LIFE AFTER MEDICAL SCHOOL

Thirty-Two Doctors Describe How
They Shaped Their Medical Careers

LEONARD LASTER, M.D.

W. W. Norton & Company
New York • London

For information about permission to reproduce selections from this book,
write to Permissions, W. W. Norton & Company, Inc., 500 Fifth Avenue,
New York, NY 10110.

The text of this book is composed in Trump Mediaeval
Composition by Bytheway Typesetting
Manufacturing by Courier Companies
Book design by Justine Burkat Trubey

Library of Congress Cataloging-in-Publication Data
Life after medical school : thirty-two doctors describe how they
    shaped their medical careers / by Leonard Laster.
        p.   cm.
    1. Medicine—Specialities and specialists.   2. Medicine—
Vocational guidance.   I. Laster, Leonard.
    R729.5.S6L53   1996
    610.69—dc20   95-5551

ISBN 0-393-71030-0

W. W. Norton & Company, Inc., 500 Fifth Avenue, New York, N.Y. 10110
http://web.wwnorton.com
W. W. Norton & Company, Ltd., 10 Coptic Street, London WC1A 1PU

    3   4   5   6   7   8   9   0

Becoming a doctor doesn't just happen by itself; it involves judicious and sometimes difficult decision making. The need to make these judgments crops up long before an evolving physician knows all that much about what life is like in the various branches of medicine or, perhaps even more important, about who he or she really is. The stories in this book convey the thoughts, emotions, expectations, and unexpected turnings that led a group of doctors to create their lives in medicine. Perhaps their experiences will help others to confront the challenge.

TABLE OF CONTENTS

PART THREE: WHICH PERSON FOR WHICH PATH? REFLECTIONS OF TRAINING PROGRAM DIRECTORS

PART FOUR: NATIONAL HEALTH POLICY — PARTICIPATING PHYSICIANS

PART FIVE: CONFRONTING OBSTACLES AND SETBACKS

THANKS

I am pleased to acknowledge my gratitude and indebtedness to several individuals and organizations for their generous help in bringing this book into being.

I have enjoyed working with W. W. Norton & Company. Thanks to Dr. Stephen Rous for originally suggesting that I write a book for medical students, to John Meyer for his encouragement and help, to Howard Boyer for his excellent editing, and to Donald Lamm for introducing me to the Norton family.

The physicians represented in the 32 stories all cooperated enthusiastically and entered into the spirit of the project without hesitation, and I thank them. Without the secretarial skills that accomplished the transfer of the interviews from voice to printed copy, there would have been no book and I gratefully acknowledge that help.

The Josiah Macy Jr. Foundation provided a grant to help defray some of the costs involved in getting the job done and I thank them. The three stories in Part 4 appeared originally in question-and-answer form in *MD Magazine* and I thank its publisher for permission to include modified versions of the interviews in this book.

Last, and most important to me, my wife and children put up with my moments of uncertainty and procrastination, provided intelligent advice and criticism, and offered words of encouragement such as, "Good grief, haven't you finished it yet?" Above all, I thank them.

PRELUDE

As a child or as a teenager, for one reason or another, you become fascinated with the idea of becoming a doctor and commit yourself to it. Then you devote much of your high school and college years to the overriding goal of getting into medical school. Once there, you find that staying in medical school demands the same intensity of effort from you that it took to make your way into it, and so, once again, you get caught up in a pressured, highly demanding day-to-day existence. Then as you start the last two years of medical school feeling the need of some serious decompression from all the earlier intensity, lo and behold, you find yourself confronting as difficult a challenge as you have yet encountered—deciding what comes next.

Life, for anyone, regardless of how you choose to spend it, presents an array of choices, decision points that have a great influence on how the rest of your story will play out. For a future doctor in the third or fourth year of medical school, the answer to "What next?" constitutes such a critical milestone, one that ranks in emotional stress with decisions about whom to marry, whether to have children and, if so, how many, where to settle down, and, in later years, how best to care for incapacitated parents.

In medicine, the "What next?" issue is structured by questions within questions and for some doctors that issue doesn't go away after residency or fellowship. Thus, you may elect to go into surgery as your first decision, but then comes the question of which field of surgery, and then of how far to go in the direction of specialization within that field, and then of which work setting to choose—academe, practice, government, industry, and so on—somewhat like the Chinese boxes within boxes.

1

None of these personal and usually solitary decisions is easy. By and large, you are pushed to begin making them so early in your professional development that you really don't know all that much about who you are and what you want in life. At that time, in all likelihood you will also know frustratingly little about the cultures of the various disciplines of medicine, about the pattern of daily life in each of them, about the personality traits of the colleagues you will meet in them, or about the influence that a lifetime spent in a certain field of medicine can have on your development as a human being. Your alternative choices are not readily plugged into any sort of mechanistic aid such as a decision tree, and so you just do the best you can and hope that in the long run the field you pick will turn out to be reasonably compatible with your inner dreams.

Some time ago, while thinking back on my own crossroads and turning points, I decided that it might be helpful to medical students to have a book of this sort available. When I started working on it, the process of making medical career decisions seemed imposing enough, but as the project neared completion, swiftly changing external factors were rendering the decision-making process more complex and intimidating than ever.

Governmental actions and cascading evolutionary changes in the private sector will modify the basic context in which medicine is practiced and taught and may well transform the underlying spirit and culture of clinical medicine. Hardly a day passes without a new proposal for a significant alteration of the economic, social, or political underpinnings of medical practice, and any one of these could distort profoundly the relationship between doctor and patient for decades to come. All this greatly complicates a medical student's career decisions.

Still, you should not permit the turbulence of these times to overshadow the spiritually attractive and intellectually absorbing attributes of life as a doctor. These will endure. Try not to allow today's unrest to deprive you of the quiet excitement that should accompany the process of crafting a medical career. No matter how the administrative and economic aspects of medical care may change, when the new laws have been signed and the new regulations have been promulgated, you will still be engaged in caring for anxious human beings who come to you fearful about their symptoms, looking for an accurate diagnosis, and hoping for a complete cure. They will turn to you for technical skill, for sincere interest in them as individuals, and for dedicated advocacy on their behalf. They will expect you to stay with them for the long haul—not just for an occasional office visit or for an individual episode of acute illness. It is from your efforts to meet such expectations that you will develop the facets of a satisfying and fulfilling life for yourself as a doctor.

To many college students who do not choose to go into medicine it appears that a premedical choice sets someone on a fixed course that virtually eliminates any more anxiety regarding what to do in life. But things are rarely what they seem, and the commitment to a premedical course only sets the stage for other difficult choices and puts them off to a later time.

For some medical students the complexities of those subsequent choices and the growing uncertainties about the future of health care in this country may generate a fanciful wish for the power to predetermine a career path early in life and thus be done with the interminable thinking and analyzing. That would not be a very good idea. It could lead to gross errors in judgment while dampening the excitement of working out your future in progressive steps. You need the beneficial influences of time, experience, and maturation to form your insights into who you really are and to enhance your understanding of the various fields of medicine. You also need time to sort out how other factors, such as societal, parental, or peer pressure, will affect your career decisions.

To some extent, arriving at a decision that works for you involves being in the right place at the right time, but that entails being able to recognize "right places" and "right times." You need to have developed your personal values fully enough to be able to assess what is right for you. You must accommodate to the reality that designing a good life in medicine means balancing reliance on care- fully reasoned action with exploitation of chance opportunity. In the end, as with other milestone decisions in life, and like the rest of us, you will probably fall back on a great deal of plain old muddling through.

All this being so, I wondered at the start, in what way could this book help? Books are available that provide data about salaries, working hours, degrees of satisfaction, and other apparently quanti- tative factors related to the specialties of medicine. Still other books contain useful descriptions of residency programs—their daily time demands, their duration, the opportunities they offer for further advancement, and the like. These books are valuable but I felt that they aren't personal enough.

As I watched my daughter go through medical school (she is now in her fourth year of residency training), I saw her interests unfold from an initial consideration of psychiatry, to a serious look at internal medicine, and finally to the selection of pediatrics, and I saw the good use she made of talks with people who had already run the gauntlet.

Although nothing substitutes fully for live conversations, a student's access to counselors and role models for long, contemplative talks is limited sharply by the demands of academic schedules and clinical duties that regiment the days of students and their advisors. So, as an adjunct to direct personal discussions, I am providing here, in somewhat conversational form, the reflections of a group of physicians about their experiences in choosing a direction in medicine.

I interviewed doctors who work in a variety of clinical fields and practice settings, who come from diverse social, cultural, and ethnic backgrounds, and who have a wide assortment of professional goals and aspirations. They all cooperated enthusiastically, enjoying both a pause for retrospective self-evaluation and a chance to help prospective doctors.

For logistical reasons, I interviewed mainly physicians who live in my section of the country. Although their stories may not reflect all the differing influences of geography, clinical work setting, and social attitudes, they nevertheless offer a wide range of observations and views.

I covered factors that lead people into certain clinical fields, into specialty areas, into medical disciplines removed from hands-on patient care, into administrative positions, and into pursuits divorced from medicine itself. I included discussions about primary care, general care, and specialty care. I also interviewed directors of residency training programs since they are responsible for evaluating candidates for the compatibility of their personalities with their chosen disciplines. I had conversations with physicians who are advising on national policy decisions that will influence the future directions of clinical medicine. You cannot fully anticipate or plan for these policy decisions, but you may wish to take them into consideration as you search for your place in tomorrow's medicine. Finally, I offer up stories about physicians who have confronted professional barriers or problems and have dealt with them in one way or another.

After conducting the interviews in question-and-answer form, I shortened and edited them into narrative texts. In trying to preserve the conversational tone, the informality, and the revelations of personality traits that made the exchanges so interesting to me, I may have intruded inadvertently on the preferred literary style of the participants. The book contains no authoritative road maps through life—they don't exist—but it does offer agreeable reading and an opportunity to sample, catch-as-catch-can, an interview here and an interview there. My own comments are intended to add relevant overviews, but in the end the interviews make up the core of this book.

If any themes emerge with consistency, they are first, be true to yourself, and second, nurture a sense of life as an adventure. As you start medical school, get past your awe at having been admitted and be aware that your decision about how you want to live your life as a physician begins when you enter medical school, if not earlier. Don't treat the first 2 years as just an extension of college course work; it is valuable time to get to know yourself and to explore the potential intellectual and spiritual breadth of a career in medicine.

During the third-year clerkships and the fourth-year electives, you get to sample the main branches of medicine. The clerkships are relatively brief, their settings vary in quality, and one of their primary academic purposes is to confer clinical knowledge and skills and to enable you to generate a record on which to qualify for a residency. As well, clerkships are opportunities to study your preceptors and to experience the culture and ambience of different medical fields—a good time for maturation and for an illuminating private journey.

In this journey of discovering what in medicine is right for you, you will be asking yourself many questions. Is it a lifelong involvement as a psychiatrist with the mental and behavioral abnormalities of human beings? Is it related to the immediate satisfaction that comes from intervening surgically and saving someone's life? Is it rooted in long-term service as a friend and a physician to chronically ill patients? Or is it associated with a sense of wonder over a profound biological phenomenon such as human vision? Your ultimate choice of a niche in medicine may grow out of a lasting childhood interest, or it may arise from understandings about yourself that you acquire later in life. Whatever field you choose, the stories in this book are intended to help to sustain and enhance your passion for clinical medicine and the joy that you will derive from it.

In planning their careers, some medical students and residents try to leave as little as possible to the vagaries of chance. They collect and analyze data and approach their decisions almost as mathematical calculations. Others make some use of data and logic but rely much more heavily on fate, fortune, people they meet along the way, and personal intuitions in their decision making. It makes the most sense to strike a proper balance between the two approaches.

A fourth-year medical student or a resident who has not yet decided what to do in medicine may feel burdened by the pressure to do so or concerned that a premature choice will constitute a permanent commitment to an incompatible way of life. The important thing to realize is that there is room for late blooming and late self-discovery. If you are nearing decision time and are still uncertain about what to do, one option is to apply to a general training program in which you can test various clinical fields before making a long-term judgment.

Among the people represented in this book, several made course corrections later in life that worked out well. With patience and perseverance an early decision that turns out to be all wrong, or even just not quite right, can be modified well into the game. After 10 years in practice, the pediatrician who cared for our children surprised my wife and me by closing his office and entering a psychiatry residency. To the best of my knowledge, it was a good move for him. Another friend trained in surgery for 5 years and then returned to the basic sciences, eventually becoming chairman of biochemistry in a medical school.

A reassuring view expressed in some of the interviews is that there is no one absolutely right decision for an individual. Several of the participants are confident that they would have been equally content with a medical discipline different from the one they chose, and feel that satisfaction and happiness come as much from within oneself as from external considerations. This may sound like a cliché, but it is worth bearing in mind.

Give consideration to the impact of outside influences on your thinking. A medical student's career plans may be guided in one direction or another by nonphysician parents trying to impose their own unfulfilled aspirations for a career in medicine on their children, by physician parents seeking to replicate themselves in their children's lives, by the attitudes and traditions of a medical school, by faculty role models endeavoring to revise their own histories in the form of a student's career, or by a patient who dies during a student's ward rotation and leaves the student with haunting feelings of personal responsibility. It is good to reflect on these pressures and give them some weight, but it would be a mistake to let them lead you to violate your character or to disregard your inner voice. It may take determination to be yourself, but it's your life and no one else's.

Not to be overlooked either is the capacity of an early brush with an illness, yours or a relative's, to influence your choice of a medical field. One of my fellow interns who as a child had undergone a splenectomy for thrombocytopenic purpura went on to become a hematologist, and a classmate who came to medical school with a nearly incapacitating limp from childhood osteomyelitis became an orthopedic surgeon with emphasis on sports medicine. Your external influences are neither good nor bad, helpful nor harmful, but simply realities to be contemplated and put to best possible use.

In anyone's life—physician or not—it is important to believe deeply in something beyond personal material gain. Medicine is not just a job by which to earn a living; it is a way of life. You would do well to enter into it guided by a lasting faith in the joy of life, in the value of compassion, or in the importance of service to others— whatever the conviction that stems from within you. To live out a medical career motivated primarily by self-seeking goals will lead one to spend life grasping at opportunities for affluence or fame as something of a spiritual chameleon, and, in all likelihood, to end one's career with a host of memories tinged by vain regrets.

Contemporary critics maintain that physicians have become too preoccupied with money, social position, or academic recognition. With exceptions, I have not found that to be generally true of the doctors I have known. The magnitude of the demands imposed by their medical studies and clinical training and the depth of the self-commitment that these require are so great that only a myopic few devalue their life work by concentrating on superficial values.

Your own vision of a successful medical career may stem from a conviction that children lend meaning to this life and that the medical care we provide for them serves as an authentic metaphor for our highest societal values. Or, your guiding vision may derive from similar feelings about the care we give to the elderly, the poverty-stricken, or the physically handicapped. Then again, you may believe that one of humanity's more admirable attributes is the irrepressible drive to fathom the inner workings of the universe and of the people in it, and that biomedical research constitutes a fundamental element of our collective quest for an understanding of the human condition. Whatever it is that you believe in, it should inform and guide your decision about what to do with the extradordinary opportunity afforded by admission to medical school.

Yet another important consideration in defining your proper role in medicine is the matter of stigma. Although, as I have just suggested, it is best to follow a dream that reaches beyond self-interest, I believe too that at the same time you should try to satisfy the needs of your nature and character. For example, you may want to become a physician and you may be well suited to the profession, but you may not really enjoy ongoing day-to-day contact with individual patients. If so, you should not feel embarrassed or even slightly disgraced by a decision to enjoy the intellectual and professional challenges of medicine while assuming responsibility for little more than the temporary management of acute clinical problems, as in emergency medicine, or while distancing yourself from direct patient care, as in pathology or radiology.

If you have talents outside of medicine and are reluctant to let them go undeveloped, there is no reason to suppress them while pursuing a career as a physician. Practicing cardiologists have written novels, obstetricians have written poetry, and the current governor of Vermont continued to conduct an active practice as a general internist while serving as a state legislator and as lieutenant governor.

Men and women in medicine who wish to enjoy the full rewards of parenthood encounter obstacles that give rise to career balancing acts. Although it is changing, women confront this dilemma more often than men and with greater intensity. Some women tough it out and stay with a demanding field of medicine no matter what the sacrifices, whereas others choose a career path more compatible with family life. Here, especially, it is important early on to free yourself of all "drop-out" guilt in planning your life. As one young woman physician who had to make a difficult career choice put it, "When you go home at night to your children, it isn't the dean of students from your old medical school or the chairman of your department in your hospital who greets you at the door, and what those people think becomes irrelevant." No one is obliged to meet expectations imposed by parents, academic mentors, supervisors, or peers.

You are not even obliged to stay in one field indefinitely. If you believe that occasional career changes will promote your intellectual growth and sustain your enthusiasm for being a doctor, bear in mind that medicine offers opportunities to experience professional life in many different directions. Although most physicians stay in one chosen field, others spend a few years in one area and then move on to another. From their earliest days in medical school some physicians set their sights on a professional goal—such as a high academic appointment, qualification in the practice of a glamorous specialty, or leadership of a professional organization—and go about their daily activities with their eyes fixed almost exclusively on that goal, whereas others follow unexpected leads and allow time, place, and fate to chart their professional course.

Even the unformed thoughts and feelings of childhood or early life deserve respectful attention. If you conclude as a college or medical student that your personality will not adapt well to a lifetime of listening to other people unburden themselves about their anxieties, unhappiness, and behavioral aberrations, you are unlikely to discover in middle age that you should have become a psychiatrist. Or, if as a youth you are aware that you have mediocre manual skills, and if you feel as a medical student or resident that the stress of putting yourself on the line every day generates more anxiety than you can tolerate, it is unlikely that you will discover after decades of practice as an internist that you should have become a cardiothoracic surgeon.

The insights of youth needn't direct you away from a field; they may draw you toward one as well. As a youngster you may find yourself to be a caring person and then discover later on as a medical student that you are endowed with the patience to cope with managing clinical problems that lie outside the boundaries of current scientific knowledge. If so, you may enjoy practicing geriatrics or caring for patients with complex or poorly understood chronic diseases such as diabetes or rheumatoid arthritis.

Your choice of a direction in medicine may be shaped by your feelings about the people who populate a certain specialty, people with whom you spend much of your daily life when you join their discipline. Your choice may also be influenced by your reactions to the hierarchical organization that characterizes a field. If you are stirred by the concept of medicine as a war against human disease, then perhaps the dramatic setting of the operating room, the style of the working relationships within the surgical team, and the gratification of achieving rapid victories will lead you into surgery.

Choosing a field of medicine begins with deciding whether you want to spend your career:

- As a physician (this category contrasts with surgery and includes pediatrics)
- As a surgeon (this includes obstetrics and gynecology, otolaryngology, and the other disciplines that involve surgical intervention)
- In psychiatry or other pursuits related to mental health
- As a physician engaged in activities that are tied to patient care but do not require much ongoing or direct contact with patients, such as anesthesiology, pathology, radiology, or nuclear medicine
- In areas that bear little if any relationship to medicine — writing fiction, composing music, managing a corporation or another type of large organization, or entering political life

The first part of the book presents stories of physicians who have gone in one or another of these five directions.

Part One

THE FIVEFOLD PATH— THE BASIC CUT

The stories in this section illustrate various aspects of picking and choosing among the five basic career directions in medicine that were listed at the end of the prelude. To illuminate these topics I sought out doctors whose histories seemed relevant and helpful, people who share similar professional attributes and exhibit common attitudes toward medicine but whose personalities and values also diverge in many subtle and not so subtle ways.

Some of these physicians entered their chosen disciplines with their professional and personal characteristics already fairly well formed. Indeed, they may have selected their disciplines because of those preexisting character traits. Others appear to have acquired their defining characteristics during their years in medicine.

As you read their histories, you would do well to sort out how these people differ from one another and how they are alike, while at the same time comparing and contrasting yourself with them. The word "doctor" covers a broad range of personalities, perspectives, capacities, and approaches to people. Envisioning whose way of life would best suit yours may help you to evaluate whom you resemble now and whom you would hope to grow to resemble as you evolve into a physician.

For some of you the choice of a category will take shape almost subconsciously with time, and for others it will derive from a deliberate decision. In either case, the choice will reflect your ethical and social values, your aspirations in life, and your personal behavioral traits, among other factors. The interviews can serve as a starting point for your probing exploration of these subjects as well as the overriding question of who you are.

Chapter 1

MEDICINE

In medicine you try to keep people well, you care for them when they are sick, and you support them through the difficult times when clinical intervention offers little hope of even delaying a negative outcome. You have to master an enormous and ever-changing body of information and utilize it in the detective work of diagnosis and the strategic work of clinical management. You also need sufficient inner resources to enable you to bring comfort, empathy, and wisdom to your interactions with your patients, and you need enthusiasm and optimism to sustain supportive relationships with patients over the long term.

Dr. Donald Girard is a general internist in the Department of Medicine at the Oregon Health Sciences University in Portland, Oregon. Until the fall of 1994, he was the head of the Division of General Medicine. Now he is head of the Division of Continuing Medical Education in the school of medicine. He is a professor of medicine and conducts an active clinical practice. I knew him when I worked at the medical center there and he was my family's doctor; now on the opposite coast, my wife and I continue to feel that he ranks among the doctors we have met along the way who exemplify well our vision of what a physician ought to be.

Donald Girard, M.D., General Internal Medicine, Academic Medical Center

I am not among those who feel that medicine has deteriorated as a way of life. It has its problems, but it is still a most honorable profession.

I grew up near Los Angeles with an identical twin brother who also became a doctor. Our father was a stoic person who suffered some significant illnesses including carcinoma of the lip and consequent disfiguring surgeries, and I was deeply affected by how he dealt with his diseases. One couldn't help but be attracted to his deep love for his family and for other people. As a result, my brother and I felt a strong need to be closely involved with people, and medicine turned out to be a way to fulfill it. In addition, we grew up under the influence of a general practitioner who focused on pediatrics and who was the epitome of the caring and knowledgeable physician. We often joined him on his Saturday rounds.

In time, we both attended Pomona College and then we went on to different medical schools. Now my brother practices obstetrics in northern California and I'm here in the Pacific Northwest. I went to Baylor Medical School where I considered every clinical rotation as a possible career choice and eliminated many of them, such as the surgical subspecialties, because they didn't involve sufficiently comprehensive attention to patient problems.

I was attracted to pediatrics because it deals with youthful patients, most of whom get well. I enjoyed working with the families of the patients and found that pediatricians and their support personnel tend to have nice personalities and to be very caring. I didn't go into pediatrics because of internal medicine.

I ought to back up and point out that at Baylor, even though surgery was the most powerful and glamorous department, I was put off during my senior year clerkship by the personality of the department chairman. He was somewhat like surgeons in general, who, stereotypically, are perceived to be decision makers who don't always listen to or hear their patients. Also, for me, surgery, despite its important contribution to medical care, was not at medicine's core. Now let me surprise you by adding that for a period I was going to be an oncologic surgeon.

As a senior medical student, I worked with an exceptionally talented cancer surgeon who was also the warmest physician I have ever met. In cancer, where sensitivities are especially important, he was fabulous and I wanted to be like him. That lasted until my internship at the University of Washington's King County Hospital in Seattle where I took a rotating internship as the first step in a surgery program.

I went to medical school during the Vietnam era with a Berry Plan military service deferment in surgery. I intended eventually to return to Houston, complete a surgical residency, and do cancer surgery. But my third internship rotation was in medicine and again I was struck by medicine's role as the core specialty where the decisions affect all the rest of clinical care, and I decided to shift out of surgery.

It's hard to know what would have happened had I gone right into a surgery internship but I suspect that eventually I would have realized that I was more comfortable in medicine. I advise students to keep an open mind even after they think they have made a firm decision. Explore who you are over and over again. Without doubt, there are similar personalities in the various specialties and, for whatever reason, they do group. A year spent reviewing your decision, if you prorate it over a practice lifetime, is a small investment in formulating long-term goals. With the general demise of the old rotating internships, if you're vacillating about what area to enter, I recommend starting with straight medicine because it offers the best foundation for whatever a person eventually does.

Of all my internship rotations, obstetrics seemed the most fun. Basically, you are working with a healthy patient population and most often it is a celebration. However, I found it to be slightly routine and somewhat limiting. If family medicine had residencies then, I might have selected it, but in the end, it came down to the intellectualism and depth of internal medicine compared to the more algorithmic approach and wider breadth of family medicine. I never considered psychiatry because I thought it lacked science. At that time I didn't appreciate the real science base in the behavioral specialties. Eliminating disciplines like pathology and radiology and other areas removed from patient care was the easiest part of my decision.

As I reflect on my 20 years in medicine, I have to say that the older I've gotten the more important my relationships with my patients have become for me. From a student's perspective it's hard to appreciate how meaningful your ties to your patients will become.

It's one thing to be heavily invested in a patient's care during an intense hospitalization or for a short time in an office setting, but sharing a long-term experience as part of a patient's life is irreplaceable. This feeling grows and deepens over the years.

Many of my colleagues who were heavily committed to primary care appear to have burned out. I don't think they lost interest in people but it became less of a priority because of the administrative and systems problems that doctors in primary care have to deal with and overcome. For some it all grows so frustrating that it becomes untenable. That has not happened to me.

After my internship, I went back to Houston, spent a year in medicine, and then came here to Oregon where I finished my residency training and became very interested in teaching, especially in resident education. Then I did 2 years of obligated military service at an army hospital in Georgia running the internal medicine area of a family practice residency program and making plans to join a former fellow resident in an internal medicine practice in Portland. But I decided that first I would spend a few more years in teaching and try out an academic position, so I accepted an appointment in this medical school.

My family and I had enjoyed the northwest but we weren't tied to it. My geographic choice was determined by the solid job offer from Oregon. In addition, my family was in California and Linda's was in Montana. Looking back, I don't think life would have turned out very different anywhere else.

Incidentally, Linda and I met in college and were married in the summer between my sophomore and junior years. We have two children. Katy, a senior in high school, is tentatively interested in medicine. John, a 1994 graduate of Stanford University, changed his career goals from law to medicine after sampling an eclectic curriculum. I encourage young people to consider medicine but I never push it. I've seen too many students who were pressured into medicine by their parents and who ended up not liking it and feeling terribly guilty about not liking it. However, I am not among those who feel that medicine has deteriorated as a way of life. It has its problems, but it is still a most honorable profession.

So I came back here and joined the faculty as director of ambulatory care at the Veterans Administration Hospital. With an old friend as my associate, I planned to develop a division of general medicine. There were only a few of them around then.

I never considered a subspecialty—it's too confining. I don't intend to be disparaging, but a subspecialist is usually not able to practice as a comprehensive physician. Because the subspecialist becomes certified in internal medicine first, many people believe that he or she is an internist as well. That may be true early on but in the long run, and with exceptions, a subspecialist cannot maintain broad medical competence. Also, general care by a subspecialist tends to be more costly because more problems are referred out.

It depends on where you work. The cardiologist in a university hospital may do 80 percent cardiology and spend much of that time in the catheterization lab. In a small city remote from an academic medical center it may be 30 percent cardiology and the rest internal medicine, and so there the specialist has a better chance of maintaining general competence. Whether a general internist can provide as good care to a patient with a heart problem as a cardiologist depends on the internist's knowledge base and his or her ability to recognize the threshold for getting help, but that is true in every field.

An internist should be able to care for about 80 percent of the diseases in most subspecialty arenas. The more complex problems do require a subspecialist. The factors that facilitate a good balance, and therefore good patient care, are collegial relationships, mutual respect, and day-to-day free and open discussion through good communication between subspecialists and internists.

After 4 years at the VA hospital, I relocated to the university because I found the administrative demands excessive and the VA bureaucracy intolerable due to the inflexibility inherent in a very large, centralized system. It did not allow for timely or constructive input from people at the local level. As we try to work out our national problems through managed care, large health maintenance organizations (HMOs), and centralized budgeting, there is some risk of replicating the same type of problems that I encountered. However, the risk is worth taking if we can do something about providing access to health care for everyone. If we create a new bureaucracy, that may undo our plans but I'm not sure we have a choice.

At the university, I entered another bureaucracy, one that was more flexible but still far from ideal. My first 2 years were awful. Almost daily, I decided to throw in the towel and go into practice, but teaching and building a program kept me going. Not that you can't do that in a practice setting too. There you can develop patient education, a system for efficient care, and preventive programs. On the faculty I enjoyed the opportunity to sample a variety of experiences and to have several themes: patient care, teaching, administration and program organization, and medical writing.

Despite the changes that are diminishing its flexibility, teaching is a more positive part of my career than ever. I am more interested in and more needy of the input of younger people. They tend to be idealistic and not yet worn down by the system. They are bright and they value the opportunity to learn from someone who is older and more experienced. I do not have encyclopedic knowledge but I can help at the bedside. The experienced internist can impart skills in history taking and physical examination and the ability to make meaningful use of clinical information without excessive reliance on the ECG, the SGOT, or other ancillary data. Too often students are drawn to the ECG to diagnose angina when the diagnosis should be made from the history.

For a time I directed the internal residency program, and that's when I became interested in the dysphoria that physicians experience during their training, a phenomenon that is not well documented. Residents go through a difficult time, especially during the internship year. They start out excited about finally fulfilling their roles as doctors but because of their lack of clinical skills they recognize very quickly that they aren't able to do what they thought they could do and because of our system they are not allowed to do some of the things that they want to do. So they become depressed.

Their administrative duties—filling out forms and tracking down laboratory data—are demanding and feel burdensome even though they are an important part of the job. The new graduate physician has a lot of book knowledge but only modest clinical skill. Becoming clinically competent takes time, energy, frustration, and much encouragement from the more senior people. Residents expect to be good quickly, and when they find out they're not they become discouraged.

What is particularly shocking to a new doctor is the discovery that the patient has become part of the problem. In traditional training settings patients mean more hard work and longer hours. Each new admission, especially a complex one, requires time and energy that the house staff may not have to give, so that at some point the patient becomes part of the problem as opposed to part of the reason for the doctor being there in the first place. Then people become disillusioned and may question their personal commitment to medicine. We studied aspects of emotional change among house staff and now that's a major interest for me.

Residency is a tumultuous time. In internal medicine the second and third years grow increasingly less so, and the residents finish up actually feeling pretty good about their experience, but along the way there are very real problems. I've published about the natural history of what happens to residents. In institutions and departments such as ours there has been increasing understanding of their difficulties and in some places this has drawn more attention and generated more empathy.

A spinoff of this concern has been my interest in physician impairment. I think that something negative happens early during training that doesn't get completely resolved. Some physicians never learn to cope well and they become impaired. I work in a program for the prevention of substance abuse by physicians.

As for how I allocate my time, I have several hundred patients for whom I provide continuity care, I supervise residents in their practices, and I attend on the inpatient services several months a year. We're moving more into the ambulatory care arena because that's where you find the patients who have sufficient longitudinal problems to be followed by the doctors.

As the hospital is turning into one big intensive care unit, teaching is becoming a problem because it slows down patient care. Patients are not in the hospital long enough to provide an opportunity to observe the natural history of a phenomenon such as a consolidating pneumonia. But residents do get to see undifferentiated patients in the ambulatory setting, and that's helpful.

An irritating aspect of my life is my difficulty controlling my time. I am my own worst enemy—I make too many commitments for talks, travel, organizational work, and the like. This is something we all face, especially residents. Although in my own training we spent long hours in the hospital, almost no one complained. It was expected then, and some people still expect it today. As I became a junior faculty member, I noticed that residents felt that it was going too far to ask them to give up everything for medicine. In a major shift, the standard is no longer "medicine above everything else." According to current thinking, young physicians should be helped to enjoy other important components of life—family, avocations, and vacations.

This means, perhaps, that medicine is not as much of a calling as it once was perceived to be, but more of a job. That may be good for the doctors; I hope it is also good for the patients. Medicine's boundaries need to extend beyond those of just another job, but should there be limits? On balance, in today's society, it's healthier to have limits for demands on the professional and not allow people to be consumed. Even with limits the profession can still be a calling, but it can't be done easily. We are all torn between responsibility to our patients and responsibility to our families and ourselves. There's the inherent conflict in setting limits while trying to fulfill the responsibilities of a calling.

The doctor–patient relationship is special and to a major degree it transcends the work hours and traditional limitations of other jobs. Patients expect that and doctors try to fulfill it. I just don't know whether you can be a truly good physician and have a truly good home life. My earliest mentor had a home life that involved patting his four kids on the head while he read the literature and his wife took care of the family. He was a great doctor but he paid a very high price and his children turned out to have significant developmental problems that took years to overcome. Now here I am telling you that one of my failures is not setting limits and, worse yet, I have no plans to change.

With regard to the economic and political changes occurring in medicine, let me comment just with respect to the role of the internist. I am interested in trying to reinstate what I feel to be an almost lost position. Right now the milieu appears favorable for doing that since almost everyone is calling for more generalists and that is precisely what the internist is. My argument is that the internist is not just a primary care physician. I don't intend that to be demeaning, but the internist is a specialist in adult medicine who provides both primary care and in-hospital secondary care. That entails serving as a consultant to physicians in other disciplines who are less well trained in adult medicine: family physicians, surgeons, surgical subspecialists, and so on.

As for the rest of my life, I would like to grow more intellectually outside of medicine than I have to this point. I have been a long-term runner but age and its consequences have slowed me down. I have been a collector in many venues, including medical history, and I have done woodworking but I still feel somewhat narrow. To a considerable degree, medicine has carried me away with it.

My advice to students who are trying to decide what to do in medicine is, and this holds for all fields in life, keep your mind and options open. Let your interests and experiences define what you do. One of my regrets is that I majored in zoology in college. Doing it over again, I would choose something outside of the biological sciences—government, English, history, or something else—because a physician becomes preoccupied by medical sciences for the rest of his or her life.

In mapping a medical career, once you decide on medicine, you should continue to maintain broad interests and test a number of arenas through your academic clinical experiences, job opportunities, mentorships, discussion groups, and so on. Not infrequently, we make decisions prematurely and we really don't have to do that. The system allows you to sample a range of experiences before decision making.

Chapter 2

SURGERY

Surgery calls on many of the same attributes as medicine, but usually only for short intervals because patient relationships tend to be of limited duration. In addition, a surgeon must be able to cope with the stress of having to solve difficult and often life-threatening problems briskly through the use of technical ingenuity, native talent, and the capacity to make good judgments.

A common stereotype relegates the surgeon to the status of disinterested craftsman and elevates the physician to the status of compassionate intellectual. As always, stereotypes fade on the stage of day-to-day existence and indeed I have found some of my more brilliant and creative colleagues among the surgeons. Another aspect of the stereotyping portrays the surgeon as an egotistical martinet and the physician as a collegial working egalitarian. You must evaluate the validity of these views for yourself.

Dr. Thomas J. Vander Salm is professor and chairman of Thoracic and Cardiac Surgery at the University of Massachusetts Medical Center in Worcester.

Thomas J. Vander Salm, M.D., Cardiothoracic Surgery, Academic Medical Center

I liked the immediacy of surgery.

As a youngster, I never wanted to be a physician—nobody in my family was a physician. I graduated as a chemical engineer from

23

Carnegie Tech, having worked summers as an engineer. Eventually I realized that I would be unhappy working for a large company, which is how many engineers start out, and I began to consider medicine.

All I knew about doctors was what I had learned from having gone to our family's physician, who happened to be a surgeon from Johns Hopkins, the medical school where I ended up. Mine was more a decision not to stay in engineering than it was to go into medicine. I never spent a great deal of time analyzing what I wanted to do or evaluating choices.

I was missing some medical school requirements so I took some extra courses in biology and language and my choice of medicine just seemed to grow on me. I knew I liked working with people but I didn't feel any great humanitarian striving. I thought it would be interesting and fulfilling. By my senior year, the decision was no longer tentative, and I interviewed at a couple of medical schools.

I didn't think too much about whether I had a particular area of medicine in mind. Although I knew better intellectually, from my exposure to our family physician I rather felt that medicine was all about surgery. During medical school I was open to a lot of things and was fascinated by almost every subject. While I was in a particular rotation, I wanted to be in that specialty. At one time or another, I wanted to be a gynecologist, an anesthesiologist, and an internist, but never a psychiatrist. I wanted to be a surgeon during numerous rotations, and I was more interested in the adult specialties than in pediatrics.

I've always been procedure-oriented and have liked to work with my hands. In addition, I've always been interested in athletics, and surgery is sort of an athletic specialty, requiring physical skill. It's ironic that the government is planning to classify us as "noncognitive" physicians. I wouldn't categorize us that way, but I do think most of us tend to be interested, if not proficient, in athletics. Surgery is a competition with yourself to be better.

You need stamina to meet the physical demands of many surgical procedures. You can't know that in medical school and only find it out as you do it. It's fairly common for some surgeons to learn after a while that they can't keep up physically, but I've never heard them express it that way. Mostly they talk about the time commitment being too great.

I liked the immediacy of surgery—the idea that you can see a problem and take care of it promptly with a definitive result and without having to linger on it for the lifetime of the patient, as an internist might have to do when treating a patient with diabetes. I found that out in the third and fourth years when we had a fairly broad exposure to various specialties and when we saw outpatients. When I went through charts, I would encounter patients with diabetes, for instance, who had been treated for years and years by the same doctor or in the same clinic.

Beyond that, I was swayed, I'm sure, by role models within surgery. Most of them were very dynamic and therefore very attractive. All of their specialties seemed like a lot of fun: orthopedic surgery (which is what I thought I wanted to do), plastic surgery, and general surgery.

Because I knew that I was going into surgery, during my clinical years I wanted to fill out missing spots in my education to which I would not have access later on, so I signed up for rotations such as gastroenterology. I also spent more time than average on the surgical rotations. I came in at odd hours and got to know some of the surgical residents. I got to know medical residents too. I would pick out one who could be most beneficial in teaching me and he'd be my mentor for a while.

None of them tried to sway me, but they did influence me. That doesn't happen in the same way today because the relationship between patient, resident, and student has changed. When I was a student, residents had their own services and were supervised only loosely by faculty. The chief resident in surgery was a virtual god who could do just about anything he wanted and was proficient enough to do so.

As a consequence, students also had greater involvement in patient care and more responsibility. We did procedures that would now be relegated to a much higher level. Today you rarely find a true ward patient. At this hospital, for instance, every patient has a staff physician. Residents play a major role in taking care of the patient but ultimately the staff physician is in charge and the level of responsibility for residents is reduced accordingly. Similarly, students don't seem to be as intimately involved in the care of patients as I had the opportunity to be as a medical student.

Another thing I liked was that surgeons didn't stand around and talk as much as the internists did. I always became extremely tired standing around just listening to people talk. That may sound paradoxical because I never got tired standing around in the operating room. I was doing something rather than just listening.

Yet another aspect of the surgical experience that I found fascinating was taking things apart and putting them back together—looking into a black box called an abdomen or a chest, and seeing what miraculous things were in it. As a kid I took things apart but back then I usually broke them and was unable to put them back together. I was always curious about what was inside things.

Most people have the technical dexterity to become a surgeon. It's not so much a matter of coordination or ability to do fine things with your hands but rather of thinking through the motions in advance. That's vital to being a surgeon and is probably underemphasized. It's also very difficult to assess it until you're actually doing surgery. If I knew of a good test, I would use it on all incoming surgical applicants and counsel them out of surgery if they failed.

When I was in the fourth year of medical school, I thought I was heading into orthopedic surgery. It fascinated me, mainly because of the wonderful tools the orthopedists had. I applied for an orthopedic residency with some time in general surgery first, and I ended up at the Mass. General for the general surgery and in a combined program there and at Boston Children's for the orthopedics.

I spent 2 years in general surgery in Boston, went back to Johns Hopkins for another 6 months of general surgery, took a 4-month vacation, and then started my orthopedic surgery residency. After about a year and a half, I found increasingly that I resented my rapid loss of skills in general surgery. Because patients who need orthopedic surgery are not usually very sick, I began to feel as if I were deficient by not being as good as I used to be in caring for sick patients. I also found that when I went to the library I would invariably head for the journals in general surgery rather than orthopedic surgery. I began to wonder about the wisdom of staying in one specialty when I was interested in a different one. I also found that I didn't like operating on bones as much as I liked operating on soft tissue, even though I liked closed orthopedics a lot, that is, setting fractures and putting on casts.

I think I had to go through all that to learn how I felt. One factor was that as a general surgery resident I was exposed to a number of outstanding faculty mentors, people of such skill, dignity, and wisdom that I never got over their influence. It's not that I didn't admire people in orthopedic surgery, but the 2 years of general surgery came first, and that's what I kept thinking about.

To make a change, my first hurdle was getting back into general surgery. Mass. General agreed, and I went back into general surgery thinking, again erroneously, that I wanted to do general and noncardiac thoracic surgery: lungs and esophagus but not heart. I wanted to do pretty much all surgery from neck to feet: vascular, general abdominal, neck, lung, and esophageal.

Finishing the chief residency qualified me for boards in both general and thoracic surgery. Then, by previous obligation, I went into the navy for almost 2 years as the surgeon on an aircraft carrier but I didn't get much chance to use my surgical skills. I usually did one vasectomy and one circumcision a day, read a lot, ate a lot, and flew on airplanes. I was there for emergencies, but we didn't have many. I spent the last part of my tour in a navy hospital where I did operate. Then I took a job in this medical center and I've been here for 16 years.

When I took this job, I started out doing general, vascular, and noncardiac thoracic surgery. At about the time that I passed the thoracic surgery boards, we were starting a cardiac surgery program here and two of us who had been residents together at the Mass. General were on the staff. Some cardiac surgeons commuted from the Mass. General in order to begin the program here, and they recruited us to help care for patients by playing intern, resident, and on-site faculty member all in one. Very soon, the responsibility shifted from us helping them to them helping us; then, all of a sudden, they were gone and the program was left in our hands.

Since I had my thoracic boards, and since I was doing cardiac surgery, even if it was almost by default, I reasoned that I might as well become a cardiac surgeon. It was as unplanned as that. I hadn't wanted to do that, but it turns out to have been a wonderful decision. Ironically, as a resident I had pretty much decided that from all of the surgical subspecialties, neurosurgery and cardiac surgery were the two that I would absolutely exclude.

It would be almost impossible to replicate that pathway today. I came here before the hospital doors opened, and the institution's history formed my own professional history. Had I gone somewhere else, I might have become a general surgeon and I probably would have been just as satisfied. I'm basically happy doing what I do, whatever it may be.

I don't believe the choices you make in medical school and early residency have to be irrevocable, nor do I believe they should be permitted to generate excessive anxiety. If you're comfortable with yourself, you'll be happy in a variety of areas once you've made the larger selection of surgery versus medicine versus psychiatry. In fact, I would make it even broader. I think a lot of internists might be happy doing surgery and vice versa. However, I would not have been as happy as an internist as I am as a surgeon.

As for what I do all day, I operate most of the day on Monday, Tuesday, and Wednesday. I get up at around 5 A.M. and swim laps. I get to work at about 6:30 A.M., make rounds on the patients, and meet with the residents to discuss patient plans for that day. At 8 A.M., I start the first of what is usually a two-case day if it's Tuesday or Wednesday, or a one-case day if it's Monday. On Mondays, surgery is followed by clinic where I see patients who have been or are scheduled to be operated on. I'm usually on call Monday nights and maybe 25 percent of the time I'll have an evening operation or some emergency.

Generally, I finish work between 4 and 8 P.M. There is time between cases for lunch and for seeing new patients and consults. Sometimes I operate on Thursday and Friday, but more often than not, on Thursdays I get caught up doing research, and on Fridays I attend to administrative matters and go to meetings such as the one you and I are having now. My research involves projects in the animal laboratory. Currently, I'm working on new ways to do mitral valve operations.

I spend more than half of my time in an operating room, one way or another. I work with residents and other associates, but a surgeon is pretty much the captain of the ship with a large crew. There are six of us in our division of cardiothoracic surgery. Although we usually operate independently, on very difficult cases we work as a two-surgeon team. The rest of the crew consists of residents, a couple of assistants, scrub nurses, anesthesiologists, and others. The operation couldn't proceed without them.

The challenges of surgery are primarily thinking challenges. It is also extremely trying, fatiguing, and wearing to be operating, not because of the time involved but because sometimes the operation doesn't go well. It's not tiring in the sense that you would be fatigued after running a race; it's tiring from the extreme emotional fatigue caused by having to think, to worry about what's going on, and to figure out how to do what has to be done. It is far from being a noncognitive specialty.

At times it can be extraordinarily stressful. If the operation goes smoothly, it's an absolute joy, but that doesn't always happen. In fact, frequently in a specialty like this the operation does not go well for one reason or another and I'm sure the stress must be taking some sort of toll on me. There are days when I would give anything to be doing something else, but when I step back and look at it from outside my fatigued self, I can't think of anything else I would prefer doing.

The actual practice of cardiac surgery, as is true of most types of surgery, is evolving all the time and that is actually one of the fun parts of it. Some of the operations we once did are no longer done. A prime example in thoracic surgery, to go back several years, is surgery for tuberculosis; it is rarely done today. In cardiac surgery, too, some operations that once were done frequently have been replaced by newer operations. On the surface that might seem threatening to a surgeon looking at short-term factors such as impact on income, but in the long run the new operations actually make practice more interesting.

There are frustrations, not so much from the practice as from the bad press we're getting, the labeling of surgical specialties as noncognitive. That originates not with the media but in the aspersions cast by the government. They are insulting. Although physicians in private practice will certainly experience marked cuts in their incomes, the really bad part of all of this is that suddenly, Congress or someone in the federal government has declared that surgeons aren't as valuable to society as they once were. That can be frustrating if you dwell on it, so I don't.

I'm always finding new things to do. I'm pretty busy outside of work too. I swim every day, read a fair amount, ski avidly but not as often as I would like, and sail. I grew up sailing; I had my own boat and was racing when I was 9 or 10 years old. Recently, a patient wrote to say that he was grateful for what I had done for him several years back and wished to reward me with something that he thought ranked equally with love, sex, and good food. I could hardly stop reading the letter after that introduction. It turned out that he wanted to treat me to flying lessons. He did so and now I fly a fair amount too. I also do a lot of fly fishing and bird hunting.

My wife and I are divorced, but we're still close in our interactions and live almost next door to each other. We have two kids, one a high school senior and one a college sophomore. They don't have the slightest idea about what they want to do in life, but I think they're pretty convinced they don't want to be physicians. I guess they feel I work too hard, and I guess I do, but I like it and find it rewarding. I do not think my work contributed to the outcome of my marriage.

As for my advice to medical students, let me return to the subject of their feeling pressured to make early and apparently irrevocable career decisions. I would caution them not to feel too pressured. In my somewhat wayward course I changed direction many times. I found that almost everything I did was interesting and rewarding. Although it may have taken me a few more years to get to where I was going than it might have taken someone else, I look on those years as valuable rather than wasted.

To become a heart surgeon today, after medical school it takes 5 years of general surgery and then 2 to 3 years of thoracic or cardiac surgery. Since ours is a 3-year cardiac program, it's a total of 8 years for our residents. During the first 5 years, a resident who has started down another career pathway could transfer into our program because we have no compunctions about accepting late bloomers.

There aren't many women in our field. I don't know if this is because the field is physically demanding or because women just tend not to choose it. It's clearly not because there's an "old boy" system. I think female medical students and residents are encouraged to go into cardiac surgery. It is time consuming and in order to do it well, if you're a woman and want to have children, you have to make some decisions as to where you're going to place your energies. I suspect it is mainly a matter of time and its allocation that keeps a lot of women out.

For a time, our exposure to blood and blood products raised concern about AIDS. That is an anxiety provoker, but not of any serious dimension, at least not for me. I try to be careful, but I think that as we become more familiar with AIDS we grow less frightened of it. Three or 4 years ago there seemed to be overwhelming fear among surgeons, but that's subsiding. There is a risk of getting AIDS if you are a surgeon or a health care worker in general, but it's pretty small.

Surgery provides the gratification of coming into a person's life and making a difference, but I do not usually have long-term relationships with patients. After I operate on a patient, I see him or her daily during the hospital stay. Then I see that patient in follow-up about a month later. Patients who have done well are referred back to their cardiologist, and I rarely see them subsequently. No, I don't have long-term relationships with most patients, and in truth, I don't miss that.

To me medicine is a continual challenge. It's a challenge to take care of patients. It's a challenge to operate on them. There's always the challenge of trying to compete with yourself to be better. It's a fascinating field because of the interesting physiology and biochemistry involved. I don't think of it on a day-to-day basis as it being an idealistic profession, but when I step back a little bit, I think it would be difficult not to view it as such. We give a lot of ourselves, our energy, our emotions, and our time to taking care of patients. Not many physicians that I know of do it for money. They do it because they like it.

Chapter 3

PSYCHIATRY

Psychiatry requires a lasting commitment to the study, analysis, and modification of human behavior. It demands intuitive perception as well as the capacity to pursue one's clinical work in the absence of as firm a base of scientific information as physicians and surgeons appear to enjoy. By and large, psychiatrists perform few technical procedures with their hands, and they probably do not experience the gratification of effecting sudden dramatic cures as often as surgeons do. Patience and optimism are among the hallmarks of a good psychiatrist. Tragic outcomes, such as young suicides, may becloud life in this clinical discipline, just as the patients who die during surgery or during the course of what should have been treatable infections trouble the memories of surgeons and physicians.

As with surgery, stereotypic attributions and supposedly hilarious jokes about psychiatrists abound. The jokes notwithstanding, psychiatrists can be a wise, caring, intelligent, and valuable source of help for patients who are sick or troubled.

Dr. Peter D. Kramer lives in Providence, Rhode Island, where he practices office psychiatry and writes. Some time after this interview his book *Listening to Prozac* was published. He holds an appointment as a clinical associate professor of psychiatry at Brown University School of Medicine.

Peter D. Kramer, M.D., Ph.D., Psychiatry and Writing

In choosing psychiatry, I saw myself eventually as having Freud's life: writing in the morning and seeing patients in the afternoon.

I'm from an immigrant New York family. My mother, a school psychologist, and my father, a pharmacist, each considered becoming a doctor. They expected me to become a lawyer; in time my younger sister did that.

I went to a public high school. Although I took extra courses in science and math, I was really more interested in the humanities. At Harvard College I majored in English history and literature, hoping to become a writer. Failing that, I thought about law, but medicine never crossed my mind. I wrote for the college newspaper and was a stringer for *Newsweek*.

As college came to an end, I felt that I had worked very hard but that I had not experienced satisfaction in proportion to my external achievements. Confused, frustrated, and unhappy about not having chosen a direction in life, I sought the services of a psychiatrist in the college's health care department. I had been awarded a scholarship to study literature and philosophy at the University of London after college, and he advised me to undergo psychoanalysis while in England.

Through him, I ended up in a lie-on-your-back-and-say-the-first-thing-that-comes-into-your-head Freudian analysis. I was the perfect made-for-psychoanalysis patient: I didn't really know anything about it; I was German–Jewish; and I had a strong conscience. I entered analysis intending to emerge a more creative writer. Instead it helped me to determine what I wanted to do in life.

Without psychoanalysis, I might not have discovered medicine and I might well have ended up as a driven, angry lawyer. I didn't use psychoanalysis as a form of medical care but rather as an avenue for discovering that I had rejected medicine almost without thinking. The analysis enabled me to recognize my empathic attributes and to decide to become a doctor and a psychiatrist. I was taken with psychiatry's wonderful intellectual history and saw appealing opportunities to help individuals and to analyze and comment on social issues.

Although today some psychiatrists still see medical students to assist them with their self-exploration and growth, that opportunity is only available to a limited extent. A related issue is whether a history of psychiatric treatment in adolescence will adversely affect someone's future career. I don't believe so, but many of the older adolescents I treat worry about that. I think the dangers of not being treated for an emotional or mental disorder far outweigh the risks of having treatment on one's record. Society is growing accustomed to its members being treated by psychiatrists. I always felt I was admitted to medical school in part because of treatment, not in spite of it.

I still love the practice of psychiatry but worry about the pressures on American medicine that make it less giving. Looking back, I'm impressed by the generosity of the psychiatrists who treated me and who took the time to teach me. Today pressures to produce money, even in an academic setting, and pressures from government and insurance companies make it harder to be generous.

I would encourage my three children to go into medicine in general, or into psychiatry in particular, only if it were a passion. Young people need passions and, luckily, late adolescence or early adulthood is a time when people have passions anyway, rightly or wrongly. Many marriages succeed through the early phases on the basis of a strong honeymoon, as do many professional choices. Any profession becomes interesting once you have put a certain amount of effort into it. At the same time, it is a leap in the dark because you don't get to experience the satisfactions until you have put a lot of work into the preliminary stages.

In choosing psychiatry, I saw myself eventually as having Freud's life: writing in the morning and seeing patients in the afternoon. I don't recall being driven by the need for a doctor's income. My alternative, academic literature and philosophy, seemed too distant from the real world.

I completed my premedical courses while in England and took the MCATs when I returned to the United States. Psychiatry was not "in" then, but, against advice from friends, during my medical school interviews I said that I was in analysis and was going to be a psychiatrist. I ended up at Harvard.

In the late 1960s, there was so much emphasis on the scientific and technical aspects of medicine that many students who might have gone into family practice or internal medicine became psychiatrists because those were the doctors they saw talking to patients. As family medicine found greater acceptance, medical practice grew more popular and fewer people went into psychiatry. Scientifically, psychiatry has become one of the most exciting specialties, largely because of new advances in neurobiology, brain pathways, recombinant DNA, the genetics of schizophrenia, and so on. But medical students are avoiding the field, I suspect because they are aware of psychiatrists' loss of clinical autonomy.

The public health obligations of psychiatry extend to suicide, violence, drug abuse, and so on, but not many people go into psychiatry looking at those concerns and students don't find many role models in public health or mental health policy. A good training program will offer some time in treating substance abuse and suicide, but, like much of medicine, psychiatry could focus more on prevention. In my opinion, public health issues and studies of brain opiate pathways are both medicine, and both are biology.

When I started medical school, I sought out a spare time situation at the Beth Israel Hospital in Boston. First I observed intake teams evaluate people referred to their psychiatry clinic; then a chief resident supervised while I saw some intake patients. Finally, a senior psychiatrist took an interest in me, and within a few months I was seeing my first case under supervision.

By the end of medical school, I had completed the equivalent of a miniresidency in psychiatry by showing up a couple of times a week. That opportunity gave me a sense of heading somewhere plus reassurance that I had some ability in the field. I recommend that all medical students try to find an interesting project that provides a taste of what being a doctor is like. It doesn't have to be in a field you've chosen for life. Medical school shouldn't be just learning a little about everything. It should also entail choosing some areas where you acquire a sense of the history, the scientific basis, and the kind of life led by the people who do the work. The field doesn't matter too much.

During medical school I also saw an analyst 4 days a week usually at 6 A.M., but sometimes during work hours. When necessary, I was not beyond telling the surgeons that I had to be excused from something because of my analytic appointment. Their jaws would drop, but I suppose they thought it would be dangerous if they said no because maybe they had a nut on their hands. Perhaps I was a little arrogant, but I felt that if a surgeon had contempt for psychoanalysis, it was his problem. Some probably thought that it was just asking too much to let a student interrupt his or her working day for personal pursuits.

Interestingly, many surgeons undergo psychotherapy. The idea that doctors are, should be expected to be, or should even want to be invulnerable is detrimental to the mental health of doctors. We are in a stressful profession, one that allows little time for contemplation and one that arouses great internal conflict and some family tension.

As I neared the end of medical school, I knew that I was going to be a psychiatrist, but I still didn't know what psychiatry really was—I saw all of its branches as offshoots of psychoanalysis. Choosing psychiatry barely defines a career. Members of my residency program became forensic specialists, geneticists, practicing psychopharmacologists, medical administrators, psychoanalysts, and biological researchers. A wonderful thing about medicine is the variety of paths it offers.

It is possible to go into psychiatry and have yet another major career choice ahead of you. You can remain medically involved by working with obstetrics or cardiology departments doing consultation liaison and joint research. One member of my residency group completed almost a second training program in medical genetics and is now an international figure in the genetics of psychiatric disorders, working not at the level of epidemiology and diagnosis, but at the level of recombinant DNA and genetic modeling.

With this richness of opportunity, choosing a residency required heavy thought. My mentor recommended Yale because it offered a broad spectrum. But because I was still having a romance with medicine, I applied for a separate medical internship before going to Yale. I got my tenth choice—at the University of Wisconsin. It turned out to be a terrific year, toward the end of which they invited me to stay on in medicine or in psychiatry. I'd never been as happy as I was there. Turning it down was hard.

When I got to Yale, I had a rough time. I started out on a neurologically based medical ward where they put me through the wringer. Because of my extensive clinical work in psychotherapy, I thought I knew everything. I learned that I did not. I came out with respect for phenomenologic, diagnostic psychiatry—looking at people and diagnoses from a medical point of view. I had to learn a new kind of psychiatry: making the right diagnosis, matching it to the right medicine, and influencing people through the ward milieu and family work. Least important were individual psychotherapy and analysis of unconscious conflict.

The goal of training a psychiatrist today is to impart the full range of modalities within psychotherapy and within the medical model, but there is so much material that the tendency is to sub-sub-specialize. In addition, when it comes to academic advancement you fare better if you're working with a system in the rat's spinal fluid rather than a system that works in human beings because the trend is toward biological psychiatry. Teaching analytic psychotherapy is relegated to voluntary faculty, if it's emphasized at all. It is kept alive by the interest of medical students and residents, but it's not where research dollars or academic appointments go, or where time is built into the training program. For the moment, however, the good training programs can still give a strong background in both.

The current reimbursement system mitigates against long-term intensive treatments, yet that is how psychiatrists traditionally learned psychotherapy. Because of the short lengths of stay and the low reimbursement for long-term care, the opportunity to see a patient over the 3 or 4 years of residency is becoming less and less available. In some programs you can become a psychiatrist without doing psychotherapy.

At Yale, I did a great deal of psychotherapy even though it was a blood-and-guts program in which I also did legal work, consultation to the medical and surgical wards, and ER work. On a long-term care ward I was deeply influenced by the chance to work closely with a young woman who was dying of severe collagen vascular disease. I saw the tremendous range of psychiatry and learned to function in many different settings. That is probably the usual program today, with the addition of geriatric training.

Yale had a specialization track and they assigned me to community psychiatry. It wasn't my choice, but I developed roots in that field and got to spend the last half year of my residency in Washington, D.C., doing public policy in mental health. I ended up as acting director of the Division of Science in the Alcohol, Drug Abuse, and Mental Health Administration, shuttling between policy people and research scientists, interpreting and translating between them. The real reason I took the assignment was to marry my fiancée, who lived there.

As I neared the end of my training, I knew less and less about where I was heading. After residency, I stayed with the Washington job for a few more years and then, concluding that I was not suited to government work, moved to a job connected with Brown Medical School in Providence, Rhode Island. I also started to write a book about my experiences in residency and about modern psychiatry. It never came to anything, but it did result in a different book 10 years later.

I saw an impending crisis in mental health care because Washington was cutting the budgets for community mental health services. Feeling that a general hospital might take up some of the slack, I joined the Rhode Island Hospital hoping to extend the work of its outpatient clinic to serve public health needs in the setting of an excellent university. We planned a combined outpatient psychiatry clinic for three of the major local hospitals. Nothing evolved as I expected, and in time I went into private practice.

I see patients, write a monthly column for psychiatrists in a national trade journal, and I am happy. I'm up to about 40 percent writing and 60 percent practice. I teach a couple of hours a week in the medical school and people, largely nonpsychiatrists such as social workers, see me privately for fee-for-service supervision. I see all kinds of patients, from adolescents up to the geriatric age group, but I'm somewhat overloaded with college and graduate students, on the one hand, and with physicians, psychiatrists, and other mental health professionals, on the other. Regrettably, I don't do analysis.

The biggest segment of my patient load involves minor depressions, minor anxiety disorders, affective disorders in general, and degrees of obsessionality. Some patients have a psychosis, schizophrenia, or a manic–depressive disorder. A small percentage of my referrals comes from the medical society. These patients are impaired physicians who suffer not so much from alcoholism or drug addiction but from problems related more to compulsiveness, sociopathy, or just plain arrogance. Some doctors develop an arrogance that pretty much borders on mental illness and that comes to the attention of their peers.

In a psychiatry practice many people get better, some after only a few sessions, but I can't be sure that it's because of what the psychiatrists do. Medicines do a lot for the more intractable cases. As in any profession, the longer you stay in psychiatry, the more your case load is enriched with people you have not cured. Sometimes it becomes important to refer people out or at least to get some consultation.

Compared to English professors and journalists, you certainly can make a good living practicing psychiatry, but it's the third least lucrative specialty in medicine and it may become less lucrative. Compared to what psychiatrists earned 10 years ago or to what surgeons make today, we're not doing all that well, but if you enjoy the field, society will find plenty for you to do and pay you for it.

I enjoy my time with patients. What's not so wonderful are the economic pressures and the third-party oversight. I do not enjoy being in a field constrained by managed care, that is, by having someone looking over my shoulder who may know little about what I do, and whose primary concern is to save money. The bad part of managed care is the intrusion on your thought processes by pressures aimed at making you a collaborator in giving the patient the least attention possible. Your overseer may be an MBA working with an associate such as a nurse practitioner or sometimes, a physician. All this intrudes on you and on your patients, and it's getting worse.

My fantasy is that eventually the administrative oversight will become so expensive that somebody will decide it's not worth the price. A likely outcome in psychiatry will be insurance policies that will simply pay for the amount of care that can be given for a fixed sum, say $500 or $1000, and do away with the administrative oversight. Then we will end up with a multilayered system in which it will be possible to continue giving old-fashioned, excellent care to people who will pay partly out-of-pocket or whom you will see at a low fee. This will create some moral tension, but I would prefer the financial constraints to the intellectual ones.

I'm glad I can earn some income from writing. At one time I derived reassurance from knowing that if necessary I could always make a living doing only psychiatry. Now the self-assurance goes in both directions; if things get too unpleasant in psychiatry, I could make some kind of a living as a writer.

My private joke is that the practice of psychiatry is so solitary that I leaven it by writing. Still, I regard the solitude as one of the great pleasures of psychiatry. On the other hand, how solitary is it to be listening to someone's intimate thoughts and interacting with that person hour after hour?

I'm on the staff of four hospitals and I do peer and utilization review and ward rounds. I supervise residents and teach part of their basic psychotherapy course. I have given undergraduate lectures for the medical students. For a while, I took part in a seminar on human values in medicine that brought together doctors, political scientists, and philosophers.

I have given talks in sociology and philosophy classes at Brown, and I show up occasionally in the creative writing program. My column gives rise to a correspondence that keeps me in touch with peers all over the country and gets me speaking invitations. I'm on a committee of the American Psychiatric Association, and I was president of the state psychiatric society. So I have extensive contacts with my colleagues and I have made it a part of my life to represent a threatened element in psychiatry, the private practitioner.

I could not restrict myself to clinical practice. There are too many opportunities for self-deception when a person just sits in the office and sees patients 50 hours a week. It is important to do something in addition that exposes you to public scrutiny and criticism. If I just sat in a chair all week, I would develop back pain and a tendency to grandiose or paranoid fantasies. Still, some people do manage to pull it off.

I like my psychiatrist colleagues. The psychiatric profession appears to be attracting very different people today and I prefer the old ones. The members of our residency group were really attached to one another. We still meet at least once a year. I think that psychiatry is much saner than it used to be and therefore duller. A certain degree of insanity is perhaps leavening for the profession. My old friends are all doing interesting work and my path is not atypical.

As you get older, rising in the pecking order starts to pall. The goal in life should be to fulfill yourself by having an outlet for your creative expression and for enhancement of your abilities. Psychiatry is a rich field with a lot to be done in it and outside it. During training, aim to expand your technical abilities and stretch yourself empathically. The choice of the setting in which to exercise your skills, whether it is a state or private hospital, an outpatient substance abuse clinic, a private practice, a forensic consultancy, or a research laboratory, should be a late decision. If you enter private practice and find that you don't enjoy it, other useful opportunities crop up, such as consulting for businesses or labor unions, working with pregnant teenagers, or improving mental health care for the elderly.

As for outlets other than practice and writing, first on my list comes marriage and children. I feel that my wife and I have a good marriage and am pleased with the way the kids are growing. It's an absolute libel that psychiatrists' children are more abnormal than others. On the whole, the children of psychiatrists are wonderful, maybe because we are less odd than we used to be, but I think the previous generation had wonderful children too. They may be less inhibited and more outspoken, but it's not a terrible fate to be a psychiatrist's child. My children may disagree. I work hard on my marriage. There's social discomfort in being a psychiatrist's spouse, but my wife deals with it well. In contrast to being married to a surgeon or a gastroenterologist, it involves less on-call time and fewer emergencies.

Psychiatric practice is exciting right now. It involves effective integration of an enormous variety of material from far more disparate sources than in the rest of medicine. It is a stimulating arena for someone capable of tolerating ambiguity in a field on the brink of great change.

Some changes will be for the better and others for the worse. Psychiatry is not a discipline to which fanaticism is foreign. But the potential is there for extraordinary breakthroughs, and these will have to be integrated into the existing knowledge. It will be unfortunate if outside forces inhibit the development of the field because in the long run it will be very inexpensive for humanity to have psychiatry evolve in a free-going, creative way. Right now, its clinical aspects and research programs are under siege. Yet society is probably smart enough not to destroy the profession. Given any breathing room at all, medicine generally, and psychiatry in particular, will be extremely fascinating over the next decade.

Chapter 4

DISCIPLINES REMOVED FROM ONGOING PATIENT CARE

Anesthesiology, Pathology, and Radiology

Some physicians choose to work in a field because they are drawn to its scientific or technological attributes or to the setting and organizational structure in which it is practiced. Quite often doctors who elect to go in this direction must adjust to a resulting disengagement from the ongoing care of individual patients. The stories in this chapter reflect a progression away from continuity of patient care, a progression that arises from the nature of the medical disciplines. Thus, the anesthesiologist in the first story cares mainly for patients when they are not awake. The pathologist, who appears in the second story, devotes the bulk of his working time to samples of patient tissues or body fluids, or to administrative tasks. Finally, the radiologist in the last story usually sees patients for single and often brief interactions, and directs much of his professional attention and interest to the rapidly changing technological foundations of his field.

Although the branches of medicine that make up this group are essential to patient care, their practitioners do not assume primary responsibility for the decisions and oversight involved in a patient's ongoing clinical management. They rarely experience the type of gratification that derives from the regular patient encounters enjoyed by clinicians who provide continuing care. Still, from time to time a doctor in one of these categories of medicine will save a patient's life as dramatically as a colleague in one of the other groups. Interestingly, even within the disciplines covered in this chapter the question arises as to how far to go in the direction of specialization.

Dr. Theodore E. Dushane is in the private practice of anesthesiology. He works in a group that is based in a voluntary teaching hospital in Ann Arbor, Michigan, and he is a clinical assistant professor of anesthesiology with the school of medicine in the University of Michigan. He also devotes some time to consulting work.

Theodore Evan Dushane, Ph.D., M.D., Anesthesiology, Private Practice

From my early days there was little doubt that I had a good head for computation and abstraction. . . . Medicine has yet to create the right working conditions to exploit the contributions people like us can make.

I was born out West when my father, who is a cardiologist, was in the Air Corps, but I was raised and went to public school in West Hartford, Connecticut. I went on to Yale College where I wound up with a BA in math and a minor in the logic part of philosophy. From my early days there was little doubt that I had a good head for computation and abstraction.

My dad went into practice in Hartford after giving up part-time research because he felt he couldn't make a living working in the catheterization lab. My only sibling, a sister, became a nurse. In high school I looked to medicine as a career, but I thought that I would combine it with mathematics or something else along the technical line. I knew that I didn't want to be a lawyer and I figured I wasn't going to be good in business. In college I applied both to medical school and to math graduate school. I couldn't decide between the two.

For medical school I applied only to Yale because I was right there, and I was admitted. Back in 1967, you could be admitted to medical school with a handshake if you had a good enough academic record. They pretty much just tried to get the brightest people they could get. That has changed with time. The whole process of admissions and the underlying social engineering that goes with it has become such an issue that in recent years some people have overtly suggested dictating to medical schools what percentage of their people should go into this or that clinical field.

Anyway, after I was admitted to medical school, I had a very frank conversation with some of my teachers in which I said that I didn't think I could handle the ambiguity and all the emphasis on memorization and factual cramming of information. I had a hunch even then that eventually the information aspect of medicine would become less important as computer technology advanced. I still believe that to be true, although I'm disappointed about how slowly it has developed. To my mind, the medical model of memorizing lists that are much better stored in and accessed from a database is incredibly out of date and almost ritualistic as opposed to educational. If instead you start off from the beginning, as they are now doing at Harvard, by going through the computer, you'll not only learn the information you need by being constantly exposed to it, but you'll also develop the skills you need to acquire new information all of the time.

What I have found in practice is that people who excelled in the memorization-and-regurgitation approach in medical school turned out to be very limited. They were the best interns from day 1 of internship but 20 years later they're no better than when they started out, and it shows. The people I tried to copy were the ones who kept learning all the time. To do that they had to invest some of their time in something besides memorization. They didn't have the standard lists at their fingertips but they've remained much more up to date. I'm particularly cognizant of that because I ended up in medical school 11 years out of synch.

In college, after thinking things over, I decided to try to integrate my various interests by going into graduate work in mathematical psychology; so I started out in a psychology program at the University of Michigan. I lasted about 2 months; I liked the math part but not the psychology part, which was too vague. At age 21 I had difficulty dealing with the ambiguities involved in the biological sciences, so I switched to the math department. I figured that I would get the technical background to do real research in medicine by getting a PhD in math and I saw the graduate work as a sojourn before going back to medicine. That was in the 1960s when there was enough money around to let students do things like that. Although I owed my parents money, I was not in massive debt, and I got support from the National Science Foundation and several fellowships, including one from the Danforth Foundation.

I went into nonlinear partial differential equations: It involves newer theory and newer applied mathematics and it is still at the cutting edge today. The nonlinear part of mathematics depends on computing and is more of an engineering field. You can narrow its ambiguities down to a very small number of topics. The kinds of medical applications that I had in mind relate to such things as neural networks and the flow of blood through a heart valve, and I was willing to devote 3 years to the PhD work. I enjoyed it because it was more computational than theoretical — and that was my level of abstraction in mathematics.

By the time I finished my degree, I was married to my sweetheart from college. We went out to Ann Arbor together from Yale and got married there. She is a teacher of the deaf and an audiologist. Before I graduated from medical school, she became a principal and administrator in deaf education. Since medical school she's been a homemaker. For a long time I felt that I had ruined her career because she didn't complete her graduate work, but that's not how she sees it.

After I earned my degree, I took my first postdoctorate job at Berkeley, a very prestigious place. Ironically, several people who later had that same position also wound up in medicine. Then life grew more complicated. It became apparent that it was going to be difficult to make a living as a teacher, and cutbacks in science were beginning. In addition, academic life seemed sort of dull. I liked having time to think, but I wanted an opportunity to work on real problems and to get into computing. The people in the mathematics department looked down their noses at computing. For these reasons, and for personal ones, I moved to a job in industry in southern California.

I worked on the targeting programs for the Minuteman Missile guidance system. It required a top secret clearance, which I have even today. I liked working with the practically unlimited resources for computing. It was a golden, hands-on, educational opportunity that I probably could not have had in any other type of environment.

I was there from 1973 to the middle of 1975. By then I had helped to increase the accuracy of the missile's guidance system and I felt I'd learned what I could learn, so I moved to a combined job with a consulting company and the Environmental Protection Agency. We stayed in southern California because my wife was in graduate school, and for the next 2 years, before I went to medical school, I was the at-home parent.

During that time I gave strong consideration to going back to medical school. I was 30 years old and felt that it was then or never. While working exclusively in the technical area, I felt that I was missing something of the human element. I realized that I would never be a bedside doctor like my dad because relating to people is not my greatest strength. I relate great to patients who understand their situation, but I have difficulty relating to patients who don't understand things. I'm also impatient with doctors who aren't quick-minded. But with all that, I missed being in a field that involved people. I knew there had to be a niche for me in medicine. I also knew that going back to medical school would not be easy but I thought myself mature enough to deal with the ambiguities. It turned out that I was, but just barely.

By then I'd also had it with the insecurities of the R&D world, where we were always subject to the whim of congressional committees and military decision boards. My personality doesn't tolerate insecurity well. Later on I found out that medicine has enough of that too, but not as much because there is always a clinical component to medicine with a genuine need for what you do. However, even that may be changing now as the scope of clinical job opportunities contracts.

The whole time I was working in industry, I taught part time at UCLA. The premedical students in my math courses were awful. They weren't very bright, and most were concerned about grades. They were caricatures of premeds—and that was sobering. The prospect of dealing with them was one of the things that held me from going back to medical school. Eventually I told myself that the really bright students wouldn't be taking my elementary calculus courses and that kids at Harvard might be brighter than kids at UCLA. To some extent that proved true and to some extent it did not.

Finally I said what the heck and decided to go on to medical school. My parents lent me the money to do it. The cost of going to medical school went up three to four times while I was in school and in training between the late 1970s and the mid-1980s. I came out with a $30,000 debt, but that was nothing compared to what it would have been had I gone through on my own. During that time my wife had to deal with my not working, with moving back East, and eventually with giving up her graduate studies.

This time around I applied to 21 schools. When I started, I called up Yale and they pointed out that I was not a biology major, that I was 31, and that I was white. They wished me well and advised me to apply to 20 more institutions besides Yale. During the application process, I had to take some premedical courses while working part time. I took organic chemistry at UCLA and had to out-memorize some very aggressive young kids. In the end, I was accepted by most of the schools I'd applied to; the choices came down to University of California at San Francisco, Harvard, and Yale. I chose Harvard because they had an integrated program with MIT called Health Sciences and Technology. I really fit in with the students and the faculty in that program even though they were an odd bunch. Kinder and gentler schools like Yale or Stanford might have been better for me from the standpoint of personality, human life experiences, and maybe even career, but I felt that Harvard and MIT were the best and that I was lucky to get in.

So at age 32, I started medical school. I had no idea what I was going to do with the MD. In school I found immediately that I liked working in intensive care units; I liked the combination of technical and hands-on medicine. From the start we were assigned advisors and began working on clinical research projects. My advisor was a cardiologist and a physicist, and I liked the kind of clinical work he did. I liked children; it was fun to hold babies and examine their ears, but it wasn't fun to contemplate that as a career. I enjoyed the technology, the things you could put on screens and the data you could manipulate. So I worked with my advisor on analyzing data— not unlike what I had been doing before medical school.

Medical school turned out to be hard. I had overestimated the memorization and book learning aspects, but I had underestimated the emotional drain. It was not so much the need to deal with the patients; I was able to do that because I was older and had worked with all kinds of people before. It was the stress of dealing with the hierarchical, almost military style of the administrative aspects of medicine—the chief resident, the senior resident, the junior resident, the intern, and so forth.

We went to seminars about the ethics of the treatment of patients in medicine. But as an older person I also paid attention to the way the junior staff was treated. I found that many more ethical problems existed in the internal workings of Harvard's academic system than between doctors and patients. I felt that most of the doctors cared a great deal about their patients and did a good job for them. But in the academic scene, I witnessed bigotry, racism, and anti-Semitic put-downs, and more. If a professor had a big enough name, or if a resident was considered enough of a hot-shot, that kind of behavior was tolerated, and a fair amount of it took place.

I had the misfortune to be a member of what I called an "unofficial and non-government-approved minority group," namely, the PhDs and research types. They were definitely kicked around and had almost none of the protection of the minority label. We were abused because we threatened people.

The fact that blacks, Asians, and women were officially labeled as minority groups didn't really seem to help them very much. It prevented overt firings and abusive treatment of that kind, but it didn't prevent a lot of the good-old-boy network activity that excludes these people from situations from which they would not otherwise be excluded. My group had the advantage of being academically capable and of being a little older, but we had disadvantages, especially with academics or clinicians who were younger than we and who were threatened by us intellectually. They would do whatever they could to assert their authority, and that made medical school hard.

I discovered that I had plenty of empathy for patients and that my problems had more to do with the medical staff than with the patients. I felt, too, that if I wanted to work with patients I would have to deal with the mores of colleagues. I was going to pursue cardiology—I guess because my dad's a cardiologist and because it was my initial exposure in medical school. Also, it seemed like the most technical area of medicine, one where there was contact with patients but the job was fundamentally technical. Nowadays anesthesiology is as close to the same combination as invasive cardiology, and what I ended up doing is not all that different, but we'll get to why I switched.

I considered cardiology, radiology, and anesthesiology, chose cardiology, and aimed for internal medicine as the first step toward cardiology. I ruled out pulmonary because it depended on thermodynamics, which I didn't like all that much. I ruled out radiology because I'm myopic. And at that point, I felt anesthesiology didn't offer as much technical possibility as cardiology. I went through the internship match and wound up in medicine at the Barnes Hospital of Washington University in St. Louis. Within a week after starting, I felt it was the wrong situation for me. Within a month, I was struggling and hated it.

I was 37 and I felt overburdened by a very hard program. It involved lots of patients and lots of data; it was a crank-out-the-patients kind of program, which I wasn't prepared to do again for another 3 years. Internal medicine reminded me of the premeds I had taught at UCLA except that the little students were now all grown up and big as life. I started thinking about how to get into something more specialized without having to spend so much time in internal medicine.

The worst professional decision that I have made was to go into internal medicine. By mutual agreement, in midyear I dropped out of the program. It cost my family a whole year of living in St. Louis, a tough place for us. If I had considered the emotional aspects more carefully, I probably never would have applied in internal medicine and I probably would have gone into anesthesiology to begin with. I guess my medical school exposure to internal medicine was insufficient to give me a realistic view of it. For my fourth-year clinical electives I had chosen only ICU rotations plus one in anesthesiology.

When I dropped out of medicine I had no other job lined up, but I got a lot of help from the anesthesiology chiefs at the Beth Israel, the Brigham, and the Mass. General in Boston. Eventually I signed up for the Mass. General program. Why anesthesiology? I had done one of my fourth-year ICU electives at the Beth Israel, and there I had met the best and the brightest professor I ever had as a medical student. He was their chair of anesthesiology, and the impression he had made greatly influenced my thinking when I decided that I was not willing to pay the dues of training in internal medicine to get into cardiology.

My family stayed in St. Louis while I went back and forth to Boston to make arrangements with the Mass. General and to buy a house. Because I hadn't finished my internship, I arranged to spend a year at a local community hospital in Boston that was also a Harvard teaching hospital. I managed to cook up an entire year of ICU medicine. I was 38 when I finished. Then I did 2 years of residency and a 1-year fellowship in cardiac anesthesiology.

The career shift worked out, but it was humbling to learn that there were areas in which I probably could not succeed because of what they entailed: the kind of intellectual activity, the volume of information required, the type of patients, and so on. Thus, when it came to internal medicine, I didn't have the tolerance for what I regarded as essentially running on a treadmill. It's hard to say which comes first, the lack of ability or the lack of interest, but the two were intermeshed negatively for me in internal medicine and positively in anesthesiology.

I knew from medical school that the major part of anesthesiology is not putting people to sleep and waking them up: the real job is being an on-line physiologist and pharmacologist in the operating room. With elaborate cases the question of being asleep is handled in 10 minutes. The rest of the typical 3- to 4-hour operation involves hemodynamic, electrophysiologic, and pulmonary monitoring and manipulation. Because of our current technological limitations we can't monitor the brain very much, but maybe someday that too will be part of the monitoring.

I am absolutely responsible for the pharmacophysiology of the patient on the table. In the old model it was the surgeon's responsibility. This realignment of roles can be an occasional source of tension now with the old-line surgeons. They have a superficial knowledge of these things—enough to get by on occasion, but not at the level of sophistication of a good anesthesiologist. The Mass. General is probably the preeminent U.S. hospital where anesthesiologists have control of the ICUs and are regarded as the intensivists in the operating room. Unfortunately, the rest of the world has not caught up to the Mass. General in that regard, and in too many places the image of the anesthesiologist remains as the flunky at the head of the table. The cardiac anesthesiologists were the best ICU doctors I saw at Harvard, yet even there it was a struggle for these excellent physicians to gain appropriate respect from the rest of the staff.

When I switched to this field, I figured I would be a cardiac anesthesiologist and work in a big place like the Mass. General. I wanted to work in the equipment area because it is in the analysis of the data that we touch on the sort of things I worked on as an engineer. Before we reach the point where computer-controlled feedback systems can take over the management of anesthesia, a lot of research has to be done because important steps are still missing. If you want to use such elements as blood pressure, cardiac output, ST segments, and even automated echocardiogram data to control the administration of pressors, depressors, vasodilators, and so forth, in theory those can be programmed, although no one has done it yet. It's relatively simple and probably will occur within 10 years, give or take 10 years, since things evolve painfully slowly in clinical medicine.

The problem with the more "anesthetic" drugs — hypnotics, drugs that decrease brain activity, barbiturates, and so forth — is the absence of a good end point to measure. With the nervous system we don't have anything analogous to blood pressure, cardiac output, ST segment, heart wave or rhythm, or whatever. When it comes to concentrations of substances in body fluids, it's the brain levels and the spinal cord levels rather than serum levels that determine the actual anesthetic properties of the drugs. So we're many more years away from having neurologic feedback controls, and there's still a need for a real anesthesiologist in the operating room.

My "ICU internship" before going to the Mass. General was the best possible preparation for anesthesiology. At the Mass. General I did the 2-year program and then a year of cardiac anesthesiology. During those years I decided that academic life was too competitive for me and that the ground rules for the competition were too nebulous. Some people were doing good research and having a fulfilled life, but although the Mass. General had the best anesthesiology department in the country, a number of attendings who were engaged in trivial activity nevertheless held high positions. I could have stayed on, but the conditions would have been no better than for anyone else. One condition was infinite devotion, and at age 42 I wasn't up to being an acolyte at the foot of the seer. I felt that my computer skills and my ideas made me unusual among physicians and that to succeed there I was going to have to pay the same dues as people who didn't have those attributes.

So I picked the job that I have now. When I started here in 1987, I thought that because I'd worked in industry before I could still pursue some of my other interests through my industrial ties. I have been able to do some of that, but there has been a significant cutback in R&D money in several of the companies for which I had hoped to work, which has made it more difficult to find assignments as a consultant.

I'm in a group of 29 private practitioners. We work mainly in our base hospital and we do some work in smaller affiliated hospitals. I come in every day and "squeeze the bag" like everyone else; but because I am in such a large group, I can spend the preponderance of my time doing cardiac cases while maintaining my general skills. The group allows its members to work different amounts of time, so if the consulting activity were to pick up, I'd be able to accommodate.

Another reason for coming here was that both of our kids are exceptionally brilliant, and we wanted to live in a place where they could be with people like themselves. In considering a number of job offers, we concluded that there was no other place as good as Ann Arbor for raising kids. By then we had lived in something like 15 states and 30 locations. This place and this job have lived up to expectations, and anesthesiology was a right choice although I might have been happy in interventional radiology, too. My original concern about my myopia as a deterrent to work in radiology was probably irrelevant. My brother-in-law is an interventional neuroradiologist and works in a setting similar to mine. He's technically oriented too and we have kind of a network of PhD–physician people. Medicine has yet to create the right working conditions to exploit the contributions people like us can make.

The man who taught me organic chemistry at UCLA went on to win the Nobel Prize. When I talked to him about my going into medicine, he was dubious. He thought that it would be hard for me to get through the clinical stuff and still have energy to do what I wanted to do. Right now what I'd want to do is to spend a couple of days a week on clinical work (I love it) and the other 3 or 4 days a week working for an R&D company like Hewlett–Packard on data analysis and on interface technology for monitoring and eventually for feedback control systems.

As for whether medicine was the right choice for me, I think so, but I don't really know because life is not a controlled experiment. I do know that my going through all this and my being in practice here has enabled my kids to come through pretty well. They're 19 and 14, and I have no idea what they are going to do—but I don't think it will be medicine.

To those highly intellectual people who do look to medicine as a career, I suggest that they not underestimate the emotional and social factors involved in these decisions. There is a tendency when one comes from an intellectual background to overemphasize the intellectual aspects with everything one does. I hasten to add that if you can find the right setting for yourself, and that means knowing yourself as well as you can, a career in medicine, with all of its problems, is worth the price of admission.

▄▄▄▄▄▄▄▄▄▄▄▄▄▄▄▄▄▄▄▄▄▄▄▄▄▄▄▄▄▄▄▄▄▄▄▄▄▄▄

Dr. Gerald Nash is chairman of the Department of Pathology at the Baystate Medical Center in Springfield, Massachusetts, and a professor of pathology at Tufts University Medical School.

Gerald Nash, M.D., Pathology, Teaching Community Hospital

Pathology turned out to be everything that I had expected. For the first time, I felt that I was dealing with the whole breadth of medicine. It was like selfishly skimming off the intellectual cream of medicine without having to be concerned with caring for patients, the part of medicine that takes so much out of a person emotionally.

From childhood, I wanted to be a doctor. I'm from a blue collar background in Cleveland where I went to an inner city high school. I was interested in the sciences, especially biology, and a counselor gave me good advice about applying to colleges. Princeton awarded me a scholarship. I went there at age 18, and I never went back to Cleveland.

Neither of my parents graduated from high school, but there are three scientists on my mother's side. Her eldest brother, one of nine children, worked his way through college, became a physician and a pharmacologist, and had a brilliant career. During the summers when I was 14 and 15 and he was the director of research for Wyeth Laboratories, I worked in his laboratory. That exposure inspired my desire to become a bioscientist.

At Princeton I did nothing but study. For my senior thesis I worked on the metamorphosis of the newt and thought seriously about getting a PhD, even though I had already been accepted into medical school. But my uncle thought that even in research an MD degree would afford me attractive opportunities. I think he was concerned that I didn't have what it takes to become more than just another plodder in the lab.

Thanks to a high school science fair project I got a job working at the end of my freshman year in college with a leading kidney disease researcher at the Babies and Children's Hospital in Cleveland. I worked for him for three summers and he served as an excellent example of a physician/scientist. He was gentle, soft-spoken, and brilliant—the kind of person you'd want treating your infant. Although he was torn between full-time science and his clinical work, my time with him left me wanting to be a physician and a scientist.

When it came time to try for medical school, I became sort of nutty. I was determined to go for the best—Harvard—even though I was not Phi Beta Kappa and my MCATs, though better than my SATs had been, were not at the very top. The interview seemed a disaster—an elderly fellow gave me a problem to solve in an area of physical chemistry I hadn't even studied yet. But my senior thesis had just been published in *Science* and somehow I got accepted. When the telegram came, I broke down and vowed never to put myself under such stress again. For 4 years I had worked for that admission without doing much of anything else. I felt it was time to start living, but at Harvard I did it again. Even so, I did avoid setting myself the goal of an internal medicine internship at the Mass. General, which in those days was at the top.

The first year at Harvard buried my idea of becoming a scientist. I realized then that my uncle had been right about medical school and that eventually I should deal with patients, not basic science. I finished the second year rather undifferentiated as an embryonic doctor. During the first two summers I had fellowships with the California Department of Public Health. In the first summer, we studied suicides in San Francisco and in the second summer we assessed the health care needs of the Native American population in northeastern California. As I became immersed in the suicide study, for a time I thought seriously about going into psychiatry, but I came away concerned about its scientific underpinnings. I concluded that as a psychiatrist I would not be able to do much more for my patients than a compassionate minister or bartender. That ruled out psychiatry.

In the second project we interviewed doctors in several rural Sierra counties. In one magnificent location I spent a day with a young general practitioner who had just graduated from Stanford at the top of his class and had decided to become a rural GP. He was the only doctor in the county, and during that day he delivered a baby, treated an acute heart attack, did an appendectomy, and then returned to his office to see a young woman who was short of breath and disoriented and who turned out to have a classic case of hyperventilation—not a pulmonary embolism as I had thought.

I decided to look into general practice, but once back at Harvard I learned that almost no one from Harvard became a GP. Then, when I served as a third-year ward clerk, I concluded that a GP had to be and do all things and that I lacked the intellectual equipment for that. So I decided to become the next closest thing, a general internist.

I never considered surgery. I didn't feel it would be satisfying intellectually. A surgeon has to solve new problems on the spot and I am a plodder, a reasoner, and a worrier—an approach that is not too compatible with surgery. I never thought about pediatrics. I just couldn't handle the trauma of dealing with sick children. I marvel at how physicians can take a family and child from an initial visit through a chronic illness or the death of the child and survive emotionally.

During a fourth-year elective in hematology I had my first positive interaction with a pathologist. I became interested in bone marrow morphology and got to know a senior pathology resident who was rotating through hematology. He had an astounding fund of knowledge. He didn't have to spend time interviewing patients. He would read the marrow, analyze the medical problem, and talk to the clinician. He had plenty of time to reflect and study, and that impressed me.

When I began to consider where to train in internal medicine, I decided not to torture myself again by trying for what I thought to be the pinnacle. During my third year, I married a classmate who was from Los Angeles and I came to love California. She was going into pediatrics and we both went to UCLA even though it was then in its infancy and was regarded in Boston as a site of eighteenth century medicine. We decided to settle in Los Angeles and have a comfortable life with clinical faculty appointments at UCLA and private practices in Beverly Hills.

As I started my internship, I knew that I wanted to become a good doctor and, perhaps, a clinical investigator. Like most interns, I had a brutal schedule and always felt exhausted, overwhelmed, and scared. I was frustrated because I didn't have enough time to study and felt I was losing the basic science. I also began to have second thoughts about the intellectual opportunities in general internal medicine. It seemed that when anything difficult came along I would send it off immediately to a subspecialist.

I even saw a negative side to interacting with patients and their families. First, it took time away from studying their diseases, and second, it generated a feeling of power that made me uncomfortable. I saw the doctor as having too much influence over fellow human beings and I was worried about being corrupted by that power. Nowadays it's much different because so many things come between a patient and a physician—government regulations, administrators, accountants, you name it. I was also bothered by the feeling that internists didn't have enough to offer. They managed their patients' illnesses and helped them to some extent, but they couldn't do much for such problems as crippling rheumatoid arthritis.

I remember one Swedish-born patient and her husband who made me question what I was really doing for people. She was in her late 70s, had crippling rheumatoid arthritis and bad heart disease, and came in with pneumonia and congestive failure. Her husband was older than she, their children were long out of the house, and they were living on their meager retirement incomes.

It should have been obvious from what they implied that she had come in to die, but I treated her pneumonia, brought her back from two cardiac arrests, put her on a ventilator with a tracheotomy, and kept running up her days of hospitalization. One night, her husband told me that they were just about out of their savings and suddenly I began to question what I was doing. We had no committees then to help decide when to code and resuscitate. She arrested again and I brought her back again. When she regained consciousness, she motioned for me to come close. I put my finger over her trachea, and she whispered, "You are going to be a wonderful doctor. You were able to bring me back. Now do something else for me." "What can I do?" I asked. She said, "Please, let me die."

I almost burst into tears. I had ruined that family economically but what had I accomplished medically? It brought back all my old feelings of inadequacy. At the same time, I wondered what was I getting intellectually from all this. I wasn't learning anything about rheumatoid arthritis so that I could do more to help my next patient. My basic science was drifting away.

Then I bumped into a Harvard classmate who had come to UCLA as a pathology intern. He told me about a patient of mine who had died 6 weeks earlier. I had gotten an autopsy permit but had been too busy to follow it up. He told me about the pituitary adenoma and the staph sepsis I had missed. Then he concluded with, "Sorry, can't talk, I'm off to the library." Amazed, I asked him how he could find library time during the working day as an intern. When he told me that he always had plenty of time to study, that was a turning point. I decided to reconsider my choice of internal medicine by taking a year's breather. Pathology was a classic way to spend that sort of time, so I went back to Boston to do it at the Mass. General while my wife finished her pediatric training there and entered their pediatric neurology program.

Pathology turned out to be everything that I had expected. For the first time, I felt that I was dealing with the whole breadth of medicine. It was like selfishly skimming off the intellectual cream of medicine without having to be concerned with caring for patients, the part of medicine that takes so much out of a person emotionally. I was even willing to give up making the front-line clinical decisions. But I did discover that pathology was no closer to science than clinical medicine was; it was just as subjective and requires just as much art.

People don't realize how much agony a pathologist goes through in rendering a diagnosis. We worry that our diagnosis of a frozen section might be invalidated by the appearance of the permanent section the following day. Many of us feel that there's a clock ticking and that if we haven't made an error yet it's going to happen one day.

I like to think of the pathologist as the physician behind the physician, but not many of my clinical colleagues agree. Still, that is part of what I came to see as the fun of pathology, that is, getting deeply involved in patient care without having to do the scut work. During my third month, the head of pathology asked whether I wanted to stay for another year and I blurted out, "Yes, of course!" The same thing happened for 3 more years in a row. By the second year, I knew that I did not want to do anything else and that's how I became a pathologist.

In those days, a typical pathology program consisted of 2 years in clinical (laboratory) pathology and 2 years in anatomic. Most individuals want to be certified in both areas so they can leave all career paths open, but some do only one. Doing only anatomic commits you to an academic career because you're unlikely to obtain a position in a community hospital. You usually combine anatomic with at least 1 year of basic science research (immunology in my day or molecular biology today) to enhance your academic opportunities.

I have never been able to fathom how some students can decide to become pathologists when they are only in the third or fourth year of medical school. They probably rule out clinical fields during their third-year rotations and turn to pathology by a process of elimination. Some don't enjoy patient contact or the anxiety of clinical decision making. Many are attracted by scientific research and go on to academic careers in which they do only enough diagnostic work to fulfill departmental obligations. Those who do no science say you can't be that much of a dilettante because the field has become too complex for someone to be a generalist in pathology. The scientists say, "Nonsense, diagnostic pathology is at best a midbrain activity and anyone can do it."

One way around this dilemma is to confine the scientist's service responsibilities to autopsies where there is far less concern about being up to date. Another way is to have the researchers subspecialize in one area of surgical pathology. Both approaches are possible, but they still take quite an effort.

The generalist–specialist issue arises not only in the academic medical center but in the community hospital setting where many of the staff clinicians are subspecialists out of fellowship programs in which they became accustomed to working with high-powered pathologists. In the community hospital they work with generalist pathologists who may be solid but not expert in any one area. The subspecialist clinician expects the pathology department to provide the level of expertise that he got during his fellowship training, and meeting that demand can be stressful for the community hospital pathologist.

In the future, greater use will be made of centers of pathology excellence, such as the Armed Forces Institute of Pathology, where consultations are requested from all over the country. Most community hospital pathologists can handle over 90 percent of the specimens they see and require outside help about once a week. It's just that we are under increasing pressure to provide the latest word because of the demands being made on clinicians, especially regarding cancer. If you don't subspecialize in pathology, you end up being a triage officer handling the simplest cases and sending the more interesting ones out to the experts for the definitive diagnoses.

I spent 2 years each training in anatomic and clinical pathology, decided that my true interest was anatomic, and took my boards only in anatomic. I was thinking of starting out in an academic center and seeing where that would lead. When my training ended, the Vietnam War was in progress and I was obligated to go into the military. I went into the army where because of some investigation on shock lung I had done during residency I was given a research position at the Institute for Surgical Research in Brooke General Hospital at Fort Sam Houston in San Antonio. There I worked on shock lung in burn patients from 1968 to 1971 while my wife set up a practice in San Antonio.

When I arrived the first topical antibacterial therapy for burn wounds had been introduced and we were beginning to see many interesting opportunistic infections. We started a study of the infections and ended up making a contribution to the care of burn patients. Early on, we saw four soldiers who had been blown out of an armored personnel carrier by a phosphorous grenade, thrown into a rice paddy, and burned. The burns were not severe enough to be life threatening and the soldiers were evacuated to San Antonio. They were showing signs of healing when two of them developed a rapidly progressive shock syndrome and died.

At autopsy we found unusual widespread lesions that looked like metastatic tumors. Eventually we identified an organism that grows in the rice paddies called *Pseudomonas pseudomallei*. It produces a disease that can run an acute fulminating course leading to death unless it is treated; or it can lead to a chronic pulmonary condition. Our patients had died of the disseminated variant. Once we identified the organism and learned what antibiotics would get at it, the clinicians were ready when the next patients came in, about 50 in the next few months. I don't think there was another death from rice paddy burns after our work, which was truly gratifying.

During those years we described several new infections of burn wounds and began to define the burn patient as an immunocompromised individual. We also were the first to describe herpes simplex infection in burn wounds with consequent death from disseminated infection. We published our findings in the *New England Journal of Medicine*. Upon instituting a program of hygienic precautions, we observed the problem diminish from a ward epidemic to a few sporadic cases. As an outgrowth of this work, I went on to describe herpes pneumonia, a condition that had been poorly delineated. Toward the end of the 3 years in Texas, I accepted an invitation to go back to the Mass. General as an assistant professor of pathology and as a staff pathologist.

I planned to follow up a project I had done as a second-year pathology resident. I had autopsied several adult patients who had died in the respiratory intensive care unit (RICU) from pulmonary insufficiency. I found unusual lung changes: hyaline membranes like those of newborns. Stimulated by reports in the literature on oxygen toxicity, we found that the oxygen getting into the lungs of the RICU patients was not 40 percent as had been assumed, but 90–100 percent, a level toxic to animals. After our results appeared in the *New England Journal of Medicine*, people started measuring inspired levels of oxygen in all ventilator patients across the country. I've never made an observation like that again, but it was a fascinating episode. So when I returned to the Mass. General, I wanted to continue with that work. First, I had to refresh my general skills because while working on burn patients I hadn't been reading out slides of tumors and other conditions. Once I was back in the routine, I enjoyed the life thoroughly. The department had many talented people whom I liked. I don't think that there is a stereotypical pathology personality. Unlike surgeons or psychiatrists, you cannot pigeonhole pathologists. Some are gregarious, some are loners.

I had many talks with our chief, our all-purpose father figure, about my long-term plans. Among other issues, it had been difficult for my wife to give up her practice in Texas and move back to Boston. After I had been on the junior staff for 4 years, our chief started preparing to retire, which meant that I faced the uncertainty that goes with having a new chairman. I knew that as a diagnostic pathologist I would never become a tenured professor, so I had to decide whether I would be satisfied with that and whether an academic salary and the responsibility for supporting my growing children would enable me to do the things that I wanted to do. I decided to look around for a place in an academically oriented hospital with a residency program, one where I would be judged as a pathologist rather than a scientist.

I found such a position at the Cedars Sinai Medical Center in California, an 1100-bed community hospital affiliated with UCLA. They needed someone interested in pulmonary pathology. Its medical staff was made up largely of doctors with community practices. The level of clinical care was superb. The pathology was done by a private, hospital-based group, and the remuneration was far better than at a medical school. I had a heavy service load, but I did not have to make excuses for being interested in patient care or for doing only clinical and not basic investigation.

I was an adjunct professor in the departments of Medicine and Pathology at UCLA and did teaching and consulting for the pulmonary medicine division. At Cedars Sinai I was director of the anatomic pathology part of the residency program and I did some clinical investigation and publishing. After 10 years, I found myself longing to catch up with basic science and I also wanted more time for teaching medical students.

Blending time for science with time for service is an unsolved problem in pathology. In the future, new technologies such as "telepathology" may change the picture. It is now possible for a pathologist in a remote area to put a slide on the microscope stage and have a television camera send the image to a centralized point where an expert reviewer can move the microscope stage around by remote control. It is expensive now, but eventually a few superspecialists will cover segments of pathology for huge geographic areas and will work wherever there is a computer, TV screen, and modem.

As I finished my 10 years in Los Angeles, I found that things were changing so rapidly that the private hospital was no longer that much more attractive financially than the university hospital. I had contributed enough to my retirement plan to put the children through college and still be able to retire comfortably. Also, I was confronted once again by the retirement of my chief, so it seemed like a good time to start looking.

My former advisor from Harvard Medical School, who had become the pathology chairman at UMass in Worcester, was looking for a director of anatomic pathology. He invited me to visit and I saw a great opportunity to build something. I also thought it would be good to work near basic science groups in a center backed by state funds. I accepted the position and, as it turned out, I went to two basic science seminars during the 6 years I worked there. As usual, regrettably little communication took place between the basic science and the service wings of the department. My expectations about state funding were equally unrealistic. Despite all that, the setting was far more stimulating than Los Angeles had been.

My work is my life. The only time I ever pursued significant outside interests and hobbies was when I was in the military and had enough time to be active academically and still engage in such activities as woodworking. The Worcester years were a period of tremendous growth. I learned how to be an administrator in a difficult environment. I improved as a pathologist because I was around people who were at the cutting edge. I got closer to medical students, and I had the satisfaction of taking a troubled service and turning it into something respected by the clinicians.

After 6 years, the time drew near for the chairman to retire, and I assumed that a new chairman would want to bring in his or her own director of anatomic pathology. I absolutely did not want to be a candidate for the chairmanship because, among other reasons, I felt that they needed someone with extensive experience and national credentials as a basic scientist. So I moved here to Springfield, Massachusetts as the chairman of a large service department, where there are no medical students to teach and no basic science work. It's twice the size of the operation I was running at UMass and encompasses anatomic plus clinical pathology. I have an opportunity for additional growth as an administrator while I try to keep up in pathology, which is growing more and more difficult. At age 54, it's possible that this may not be my last job. I have always admired the ability of people to make moves. At some point I would like to do something more than fostering my personal career. This may sound odd, but during the last 5 or 10 years of my career, I would like to do something such as working in a developing country for the World Health Organization.

As I look back on my career, I have no regrets. I have contributed to the care of individual patients and to the advancement of patient care generally. I have no reservations about recommending a career in medicine. Even with the economic and organizational uncertainties that lie ahead, I still think it's the finest career anyone can pursue. Being a physician is a wonderful adventure.

Dr. David Phillips is the director of vascular and interventional radiology and an associate professor of radiology in the school of medicine at the University of Massachusetts Medical Center, Worcester. He devotes the bulk of his time to his clinical work.

David Phillips, M.D., Interventional Radiology, Academic Medical Center

We are a technology-driven discipline, which is ironic because I didn't want to go into engineering when I gave it a try. To my way of thinking right now I have the best of all worlds. Patients seem to trust me, and I'm good at connecting with them real quick. That seems to be enough for me and for them.

I grew up in Quitman, Mississippi, a town of about 1500. When I was about 6 years old, I asked my mother what she thought was the best profession in America and she said medicine. That clinched it for me. She was an elementary school teacher and my father a Methodist minister. My mother finished her college degree when I was in medical school. For most of her teaching career she worked in a segregated system, but she lived to teach in an integrated one, 10 years after she got her college degree. I have three sisters: a homemaker, a nurse, and a school teacher with a master's degree in business.

I went to undergraduate college at Alcorn A&M in Lorman, Mississippi, and majored in chemistry. After college I taught high school sciences in Quitman while I tried to figure out how to pay my way through medical school. I met my wife while I was a student teacher. She was a teacher and out of college 1 year ahead of me. We were married 2 years later. In all, it was 6 years before I started my medical education. I even spent time trying out an engineering course.

Then, fortunately for me, I learned that the State of Mississippi had a program in which they subsidized blacks to go to a medical school outside the state. I felt it was done just to keep us from applying to "Old Miss." I was under the impression that you had to go to a black medical school such as Meharry or Howard, so I opted for Meharry because I knew people there. The state paid my tuition and gave me a stipend of $1500 a year for room and board. Because I had no role models to follow, I was paving my own way. When I started at Meharry in 1965 I didn't have a clue about what I wanted to do in medicine; I just wanted to get through medical school. It was tough getting in and staying in.

About a month after I started medical school, my wife died from what appeared to be massive pulmonary emboli related to birth control pills. It happened while I was in school and she was living back home in Jackson, Mississippi, with our 2-year-old daughter. I was called one night and was told that my wife was dead. I stayed on in school, but I just sort of hung around and didn't finish the year. My mother-in-law took care of the baby in Jackson.

I got through the experience, but I was not attuned to emotional trauma. Friends told me that I had nightmares, but I wasn't aware of it. I was so hell bent on getting through medical school that nothing else seemed as important. I married again 2 years later. My first daughter grew up in Mississippi with my first wife's mother and with my family. She is married now. I had two more daughters with my second wife.

By the beginning of what would have been my second year in medical school I got back into the swing of things and was on my way. During my clinical years as a medical student, it wasn't clear to me what I wanted to do. I knew that I didn't want to enter the field of psychiatry and probably not medicine either because I found the outcomes of the geriatrics part of medicine depressing. I wanted to make up my mind once I got into an environment where I could become interested in pursuing a specialty. I didn't want to stay at Meharry; I wanted to find an internship where I could get a better handle on some of the specialties before committing myself. At that stage I wasn't dealing with finding the best residency, fellowship, or such. I was just trying to sort out what I wanted to do, what got the juices going, and what made me feel good when I did it.

In the third-year clerkships you're so busy trying to make sure you're seeing and doing all the right things that it's difficult to focus on anything else. I decided to try for a rotating internship. If that hadn't been available, I would have taken a surgical internship. I'm sure I would have gone toward something surgical because I liked coming to a conclusion about a problem by getting in and doing something that might make a difference. I thought of medical people as being like Sherlock Holmes, very much into solving the problem or coming up with the idea for the solution. Then they had to ask the guys in the blue coats to go and get the outlaw. I was more like the blue-coat guys.

I guess I have a surgical personality. My background probably kept me from being in touch with that idea because when I grew up in the South kids were to be seen and not heard. To be aggressive and black could create problems for you, but surgeons have to be aggressive. I recognized that if I were going to survive, I would have to learn how to be aggressive. Without role models, I had to learn it on my own—and I'm still learning.

In my last year of medical school, I applied for a rotating internship at Detroit General Hospital. Since people were asking me to commit to a particular field, I decided that if I had to do so, I would choose the surgical part of ophthalmology. I had observed the chief of ophthalmology at Meharry. He had the reputation of being very tough and stern, but I thought he was polished and articulate, and he had integrity. I was impressed.

I hadn't done much traveling, but cities intrigued me. I had relatives in Detroit so I applied to Detroit General, a city hospital that was the major teaching hospital for Wayne State University. They offered me a rotating internship and an ophthalmology residency. I got there and I was thoroughly excited by it all, but the work was hard and getting through the year was yet another challenge. During the 4 months of the medicine rotation, the supervision was poor. I worked on a ward with 30–40 patients, and for 1 month I never saw my chief resident. No one knew where he was. But I was a survivor. Every time my beeper went off I said to myself, "I hope that I'll have the knowledge to handle the situation or triage it in the right direction," and it worked out. Most of the patients were indigent and many were elderly. They'd have pneumonias and they'd be in congestive heart failure. I counted the days till I was off medicine.

When I moved on to surgery, the most emphasized factor was behavior at grand rounds. The chairman of the department was from South Africa. The discipline and the ranking of people was very military and I didn't like it, but at least it had structure to it. You knew what you were responsible for and what was expected of you. And you could see a level of achievement. As I went along, I didn't see much of the ophthalmologists, but despite my understanding that ophthalmology was not as strenuous as general and thoracic surgery, I pictured in my mind that it would involve fine and delicate surgery. I became concerned that I would not be facile enough to do that kind of surgery. At that point I decided I did not wish to pursue a career in ophthalmology. That happened around January. I spoke to the ophthalmology chairman who didn't particularly know me other than making the initial commitment to my residency. When I told him I didn't think I wanted to do ophthalmology for the rest of my life, he released me.

I had been observing the radiologists at work and decided to see if radiology was right for me. Every time I looked around I was in the radiology department and I came to realize that we weren't making many decisions without talking to a radiologist. They made a real contribution to patient care, but they saw patients only briefly and then moved on. They appeared to be consultants to other doctors.

My work on patients with burns and other problems of that nature left me feeling that doing that every day wouldn't be fun. The procedures got to be so routine you could almost do them in your sleep. I did feel that taking out a gallbladder was heady stuff, but I watched the guys walk around the hospital every night at 2 A.M. and I didn't want to do that for the rest of my life. I wanted to do something that would turn me on, that I could do well, and that would not be a burden. The mystique of radiology attracted me.

I made my decision in January or February when the matching program was underway. It was the middle of the year, I hadn't been at the top of my class in medical school, and I felt that I would do best to stay out of the match, scout out the top programs, and apply directly to them. A radiologist friend in town gave me the names of some of the best programs and I started making phone calls. I reached the chairman at the University of California in San Francisco and he turned out to be one of the nicest gentlemen I could imagine. I didn't know anything about the University of California, but he took a lot of time with me. He advised me to look to the East because there were a lot more medical schools and hospitals there. He gave me names of people at the Harvard hospitals and some others in New York, and I sent out about 50 letters.

About 2 weeks before the end of my internship, I got a letter from the Beth Israel Hospital in Boston and another one from a hospital in New York. I was working so hard and was so tired that I put the letters away after barely reading them. Later the New York people called me, and before taking the call I ran to my room and read the letters again. The one from Boston had the name "Harvard" on it, so I called the Beth Israel and spoke to the radiology chairman. He said that there was no time for him to go through grades or anything like that, but that if I gave him three references, and if they supported me well enough to be accepted into the Harvard system, there was a job for me. He called me back about 3 or 4 hours later and told me how lucky I was because I could come to Harvard. Then the people from New York called again and offered me a job with them. I had a dilemma because I didn't know anything about the great "Harvard system," so I called my radiologist friend who told me that I couldn't go wrong with the Harvard name behind me. And that is how I got my radiology residency about 2 weeks before the end of my internship.

I entered a 3-year training program. It was my first time in the Northeast. The initial shock was the difference in rent. I liked the thought of being around an institution that considered itself to be one of the best in the world. I liked doing diagnostic radiology, but I started wondering if I would enjoy reading chest X-rays for the rest of my life. I liked the radiology part but didn't feel embraced by the medical profession, some of whom seemed to regard radiologists as a necessary evil. I was prepared to live with that, but then I discovered angiography. People were doing arteriograms, and new therapeutic concepts were appearing. Thus, we had begun to treat gastrointestinal bleeding by placing catheters in mesenteric blood vessels and giving vasopressors.

There was a very meticulous interventional radiologist at the Beth Israel. I hung around him and kept my mouth shut. Because I didn't ask directly, he didn't realize that he was my mentor. I liked what he was doing. So at the end of my radiology residency, instead of looking for a job as a general radiologist, I decided to take additional training and stay on in an academic environment. The thought of going into private practice didn't excite me.

I told my department chairman that I wanted to do angiography. He suggested that I call the people at the Mass. General. When I interviewed there, they accepted me for a 1-year fellowship. Ninety percent of it was diagnostic; the rest involved selective catheterization to stop bleeding. I became a specialist within radiology. When I looked at a chest X-ray or an intravenous pyelogram, it was more as a clinician than as a radiologist. I didn't do routine readings. To work as an interventional radiologist, I had to stay in an academic center. I knew I would have to do research, but that didn't phase me because I'd seen what people were doing. Most of it was clinical work and there was some animal work as well. It involved trying out new media and different techniques, looking at physiologic phenomena, and things like that. It also involved a great deal of new technology. As my fellowship came to an end, I decided to stay in New England if possible.

I was offered a job at the Brigham and Women's Hospital where they did cardiac angiography. It seemed exciting. Since I had mastered most of what they could throw at me at the Mass. General, they let me off a month ahead of time to go to the Brigham to do cardiac catheterizations. I became a cardiovascular radiology fellow for 4 months. To this day I am grateful to the people there for having carved out that little niche for me. After 4 or 5 months, I became a staff member. And that's how my career took off.

I stayed at the Brigham for 3 years and got an academic promotion. Then the new chief at the University of Massachusetts Medical Center (UMass) surfaced. He was moving from the Brigham to UMass, needed an interventional radiologist to go with him, and asked me to be that person. UMass looked like a good opportunity so I moved in 1981, and have been here ever since.

I haven't done enough research and despite being tenured, I am still an associate professor. I would like to try for my professorship. It requires being more prolific in writing and I'll do it. It's ego, absolutely. At the moment I'm doing too much clinical work, but I love interventional radiology. I guess this program could be more supportive academically, but I think I'm in the right place.

As for the future of this field, it's exciting and growing rapidly. There are turf issues and the leadership needs to step in because relying on the survival of the fittest is not the way to resolve such problems. People who like being interventionalists don't all have to come through radiology. They could come from surgery, medicine, or any of the specialties. The interventional radiologists will have to be more involved in the clinical management of patients. Right now I'm sure my chairman would have trouble trying to fit all that into a program that is short on personnel.

We are a technology-driven discipline, which is ironic because I didn't want to go into engineering when I gave it a try. To my way of thinking right now I have the best of all worlds. Patients seem to trust me, and I'm good at quickly connecting with them. That seems to be enough for me and for them. Patients usually remember me in kind ways. I've been remembered in unkind ways as well, and I probably deserved it, but mostly I'm remembered kindly. For what I have to do I give 100 percent, and I've found the specialty that I like.

My sister's son is trying to get into medical school now, and I tell him I think medicine is a good career. But—and it's truer today than when I went into it—you have to make sure that it's what you want and that you're going into it because you love it rather than going into it to make money. A general feeling in today's world is that you need to be driven by a monetary motivation. That's what I worry about in medicine these days. Probably one reason for my liking the academic environment is that it is the closest thing to a place where money is not the driving force. But then, power and position creep into the picture.

If I had advice for someone embarking on any career, I'd simply say the greatest attribute you could have is the willingness to sacrifice and work hard for what you believe in. As long as you have that willingness, what you hope for is likely to happen. I truly believe that.

Chapter 5

PURSUITS DISTANCED FROM CLINICAL MEDICINE

Corporate CEO and Foundation President

By planning or circumstance, some physicians find themselves removed not just from direct interaction with patients but from medicine itself. Examples include doctors who have become academic administrators, such as university presidents; corporate executives, such as CEOs of pharmaceutical companies; creative artists, such as novelists, dramatists, song composers, and screenwriters; television personalities, such as talk show hosts; and politicians, such as state governors. When they look back, the physicians who take this path may wonder whether it made sense for them to devote so many years to their medical studies and, in many cases, to residency training. Society, too, may question whether it was right for these individuals to occupy medical school spaces that were denied to others. Who can say? For some doctors in this group medical school certainly provided them with a deeper understanding of the scientific foundations of medicine and heightened their sensitivity to human needs and concerns.

Dr. P. Roy Vagelos is an example of a physician whose interests evolved from clinical medicine to basic biomedical research. Eventually, he became the chief executive officer and chairman of one of the world's largest pharmaceutical corporations, and in 1994 he retired from the company.

P. Roy Vagelos, M.D., Corporate CEO

My parents never could figure out why I didn't go into prac-
tice and take care of patients. . . . Change is very important
to me. As things go well and become routine, my anxiety
builds and I want to do something new.

I grew up in Rahway, New Jersey, where our family had a small restaurant near the Merck Laboratories. I became expert at making sandwiches. Most of our restaurant customers were Merck scientists, and knowing them led me to the University of Pennsylvania where I studied chemistry. The school had a good reputation, it was near enough home to allow me to continue working in the restaurant, and I was awarded a scholarship.

I didn't think I was destined to do great things in chemistry because I felt that I didn't measure up to a genius 1 year behind me in high school who later became the youngest professor of chemistry in the history of Columbia University. Knowing him influenced my decision to go to medical school. During my first 2 years at Penn I took primarily chemistry courses, but during the second year I started thinking about medical school and took summer premedical courses. Eventually I made my way into Columbia's College of Physicians and Surgeons.

In college, I was strongly influenced by a professor who was teaching about the mechanisms of organic reactions before anyone else. There was no textbook; he wrote it as he taught the course. I had so much fun that when I got to medical school I hated the massive memorization and loved biochemistry because I was prepared to work out the mechanisms of enzyme reactions rather than simply memorizing them. Even so, the more I got into the clinical work the more certain I became that I wanted to practice medicine. I felt too clumsy for surgery and was too wrapped up in chemistry to believe in the hocus-pocus of psychiatry. Pathology seemed interesting, but once I got into clinical medicine I found that I liked taking care of patients. So I finished school headed for internal medicine.

The most dominant professor at Columbia made it clear that all other fields were subservient to internal medicine. He also put down everybody else, including students and me. It was terrible the way he frightened people, especially the female students, but in spite of that he conveyed the deep excitement of internal medicine.

I did trivial research in medical school. I wrote to Merck Laboratories in search of a job between the first and second years and I got a summer job working in a pharmacology laboratory for a physician who had become a laboratory scientist. It was a convenient place to cool off. I had almost quit medical school in the middle of the first year because I could not stand anatomy. During Christmas vacation, I stewed over whether to go back for the final exam. In the end, I did and squeaked by with a B—.

I finished school and was admitted to the Mass. General in internal medicine. They took few outsiders then, and it was obvious that my admission was engineered by my medicine professor. I was on his rounds one day, the only fourth-year student there, and he had his usual group of third-year students plus some foreign dignitaries. He asked how long after an infection with hemolytic *Streptococcus* one gets acute glomerulonephritis. None of the third-year students knew, so he said, "OK, Vagelos, tell them." I said that I didn't know, and he turned to the dignitaries and said, "This man is going to go to Mass. General and he doesn't even know the incubation period of acute glomerulonephritis!" He embarrassed me to hell, but that was how I learned that I was going to the Mass. General 2 weeks before anybody was supposed to know.

After a year and a half of house staff training, I loved clinical medicine. Our group had fantastic doctors. One went on to win a Nobel Prize and one is the dean of a top medical school. At the end of our first year, several doctors decided to take PhDs at Rockefeller University. I argued strenuously that they were so well trained clinically they should leave basic research to others.

I planned to do cardiology because cardiologists take care of acutely ill patients and look after them for long periods afterward. In addition, their technology is interesting; echocardiography and catheterization were just evolving. But because a military doctor draft was in effect, I had to go into the service first. I was inducted into the army, but quite by chance a head nurse at the Mass. General told me about her physician fiancé who was serving his military time at the National Institutes of Health (NIH) in Bethesda, Maryland, and she arranged for me to visit him there.

In Bethesda I met Earl Stadtman, who told me about his work on fatty acid metabolism and on esters of coenzyme A. That struck a chord. In medical school I had liked biochemistry best, and there Earl was in the forefront of enzymology. The NIH transferred me out of the army and I went to work in his lab. Even so, he was hesitant about diverting me from clinical medicine and every week asked me whether I wanted to go back.

My experience at the NIH changed the direction of my whole life. It taught me to be flexible, to do what interests me when I have the chance, and not to be afraid even if I feel unprepared. I was certainly not prepared to work with Earl. I didn't even know how to operate the instruments in his lab. Within hours after starting, though, I was carrying out enzymatic reactions and purifying enzymes.

Earl was the best teacher at the NIH and I worked with him during my 2 obligated years—half time in the lab and half time on clinical assignments. It was pure chance but things clicked. He gave me a project that was already working well. He had found a new bacterial enzyme involved in the metabolism of short-chain fatty acids, and he set me to work purifying the enzyme and identifying its reaction product. The work went beautifully.

Toward the end of the second year, I was invited back to the Mass. General, but Earl asked me to stay on for another year. He was going away on a sabbatical and wanted me to head his lab, watch over his projects, supervise several PhD postdocs, and teach his course at the NIH. I accepted, and once again the year went extremely well. On my own, I became involved in the mechanism of fatty acid biosynthesis.

When Earl returned, he gave me so much independence that he practically stopped talking to me. I found an unknown compound, followed it up, and suddenly I was in the middle of an exciting field. I stayed on for 10 years. After about 5 years, I stopped doing clinical work—I had found where I fit best. It was the late 1950s and early 1960s, and enzymology and biochemistry were what molecular biology was to become 15 years later. People were pouring into the field, and the future seemed to be forever.

My involvement had come about because the doctor draft had pointed me to the NIH. Today there is no such pressure on doctors to take time off from clinical work, and it's much more difficult to get drawn into lab research. University research departments have expanded enormously, and funds are available if people want to take time off for research. But they're pulled in other directions because the technology of clinical medicine has become so much more complicated and the training takes so much longer.

Not long ago, after giving a lecture, I walked though the biomedical departments of a midwestern university and was struck by the subdued, even depressed mood. The students were hearing how faculty have to spend inordinate amounts of time trying to get grants, how difficult it has become to succeed, and how schools are letting faculty go and freezing salaries. The labs were falling apart for lack of renovation for 20 years. That is quite different from my time as a young postdoc, when it looked as though biomedical research was going to grow indefinitely.

Returning to my days at the NIH, I was busy developing an enormous group and making an international reputation, but there was a separation between those who did clinical work and those who did basic research without considering its application to human disease. My world had become distant from clinical contact and it began to bother me. I wanted to get back to the care of patients, and I wanted to put myself in a milieu where everybody was thinking about patients. I have never come to regard my medical school studies and house staff training years as a wasted diversion. So when I was invited in 1966 to go to Washington University's medical school as Carl Cori's successor, I felt that teaching medical students would rekindle my interest in clinical medicine and I agreed to become chairman of biochemistry.

I used biochemistry to teach about diseases. We got the students to appreciate that understanding chemical reactions would permit them to understand diseases, and our course was well received. We talked about diabetes, atherosclerosis, and obesity in terms of how fatty acids and cholesterol are made and regulated. Many of the people we trained ended up in clinical departments, which gave me contacts even though I didn't see patients again.

At the end of 9 years, all of the preclinical departments were put under my direction. We also began to recruit medical school faculty to teach the college undergraduates and eventually we formed the Division of Biological Sciences and Medicine where our teaching spread across all of the university's departments. That program continues today. I also started an MD–PhD program and a black students program. I've always taken an interest in education.

I began to receive job offers, and out of the blue I was called by the man at Merck in whose laboratory I had worked as a student. He asked whether I would like to serve as head of their research laboratories. I said that I was not interested, but he cleverly mentioned that since my parents still lived near Merck I might appreciate a free trip to Rahway to visit them.

During the visit, I started thinking that drug discovery research might be a new challenge, one that would allow me to go on doing basic research without worrying about administrative work. I found that although Merck's research was good, they were doing traditional pharmaceutical industrial research and not biochemical work. That excited me because I thought that my use of biochemistry and enzymology in drug discovery might introduce a new dimension to these folks. I knew I would enjoy trying to use biochemistry to do something about human disease. But it was a risky prospect for both Merck and me. I had no idea whether I would like drug discovery and Merck had no idea whether I would be successful at it.

In January of 1975, I decided to accept the new challenge. Besides, our parents were in their 80s and we had lived away from them for 19 years. I was attracted by the chance to lead about 1500 people in search of cures for human disease. I was to head basic research in the discovery unit for a year and then become head of all research. I brought with me several postdocs and the man who had been my associate in the lab since 1958. Within 2 years I turned my own lab work over to him. There was a lot to do, but it was all science since I had someone to cover the administration.

In my first year in the laboratory, we started work on our new drug for treating benign prostatic enlargement. Other ideas that came during my leadership of the research programs included a drug for hypertension and congestive heart failure and the hepatitis B vaccine. This kind of direct scientific involvement was the greatest pleasure of my life—relating chemistry and medicine, and then ultimately affecting lives. Just think what the hepatitis B vaccine is going to do. In China the number one cause of death in adult males is primary liver cancer caused by hepatitis B and now we can produce enough vaccine to immunize all the newborns of China. We will eliminate the number one cause of death in males.

When we started, our vaccine guru was isolating the surface antigen of the hepatitis B virus from blood plasma. That was dangerous work because we had live virus all around us. In addition, we realized later when AIDS was discovered that the blood plasma came from people at high risk for the HIV virus. At the same time, recombinant technology was coming into use and eventually we put the gene for the hepatitis B antigen into yeast and made the antigen for the vaccine without having to use human blood as the starting material. Because of the molecular technology, now there's no exposure of the workers to the virus and the antigen can be produced in large amounts.

I thought that as the molecular biology of the AIDS virus was being elucidated we were doing great things in that field too. Our group identified, isolated, and crystallized one of the key enzymes of the virus, the protease, and I thought that it would take only a few years to develop a good inhibitor for that protease. But it's taken longer because the virus keeps mutating. I still think we can do it. It won't be a cure, but it will keep the virus quiescent in the cell so that the patient will not be sick.

I directed the labs for 10 years and loved it. I recruited a potential successor and, because it's my nature, I planned to go on to something different, at Merck or somewhere else. Change is very important to me. As things go well and become routine, my anxiety builds and I want to do something new.

Then, toward the end of my decade in the lab, I was made executive vice president with some business units under me, and in 1985 I was made chief executive officer. Some people wondered how a medical scientist could take over a large business organization, but as I saw it marketing and sales are simply an extension of what you know about medicines and diseases, and I felt that I could help a lot in characterizing our drugs. I saw manufacturing as an extension of what I knew about chemistry. We have terrific people in finance, which I still don't understand, and we have excellent lawyers. So, with wonderful expertise in the areas where I am weak, I have focused on marketing, sales, and production and left staff things to people who are proficient at it.

I gave my successor absolute free rein in the laboratory but I stayed involved clinically. I like to know the directions of our programs, but he selects all the areas of research. Running an organization, whether it's an entire medical school, a department, or a research group, requires working through people and with people. You select top talent, ensure that you can express yourself through them, and then you back off. I have developed a team of senior people at Merck who are excellent and independent.

I could retire from Merck at any time and change careers, and I'm thinking about what I'm going to do next. I wouldn't want to do something like being a university president, but I do think about going back to clinical medicine. I have been offered the opportunity to administer a big organization, and I probably would be pretty good at it, but I would prefer to do something that interests me while allowing me to make a meaningful and unique contribution. I haven't yet identified my next niche.

As I look back, I never thought I would go the way I did. I grew up in Rahway, a stone's throw from Merck, and never thought I would return. The lesson is to do what interests you and what's fun. I've had fun in every phase of my work.

Among my fellow interns, I was an extremely able doctor, but I do not regret leaving clinical medicine. I do not think that I could have contributed more to medicine if I had gone into practice. Valuable new medicines will become available. For example, a far-out possible application of one of our new drugs is reducing the incidence of cancer of the prostate. The National Cancer Institute is considering a 10-year, 20,000-patient study to test that hypothesis. If it were to turn out to be true, that would be a major accomplishment. Of course, all this contrasts with my parents' view of things. They never could figure out why I didn't go into practice and take care of patients.

My advice to the young people who may read this is to do what is exciting and to keep in mind how flexible a career is by virtue of one's medical training. Doctors have a vast knowledge of the human body and the biology of medicine, and they can turn that to clinical care, research, or even the challenges of running the medical system of the United States. Despite the problems confronting us today, people will always want better health, and it will continue to be a wonderful growth area. In research, what with problems like Alzheimer's disease and cancer there is no end to the challenge. In clinical work, what you can accomplish for patients today is so much better than what we could do in the mid-1950s. Don't ever let yourself feel trapped in a rut—and never become just another worker instead of someone who is doing things that are almost magical.

Dr. Steven A. Schroeder is a general internist who became interested in issues related to health care policy and who was eventually appointed President of the Robert Wood Johnson Foundation in Princeton, New Jersey. The interview with him took place not too long after he started work in that job.

Steven A. Schroeder, M.D., Foundation President

You don't know what is going to happen and you don't know what you are going to be like. . . . One of the wonderful aspects of a career in medicine is that although there are many different paths to choose, very often those paths interconnect.

I am an only child. My father was in the labor movement and my mother was a teacher. They wanted to rectify society's injustices and make a difference. I grew up in the Bay area of California, graduated from high school at age 16, and went to Stanford.

In high school and early college during the late 1950s I became fascinated with the study of human behavior and considered clinical psychology but felt that I would have more options as a psychiatrist. Although I didn't enjoy the sciences as much as liberal arts, I backed into medicine thinking that I would get through medical school and a psychiatry residency and then the fun would start.

I majored in psychology and was lucky enough to get into the honors program. I wasn't a very disciplined student in those days. I stumbled through biology and physics, and a good memory got me through chemistry. To my surprise, I got into Harvard Medical School. The time at Harvard changed my life. Growing up in California was mostly sports and social activity. My Stanford schoolmates were bright but not especially intellectual. In contrast, the people I met in medical school were quite varied and many were genuine intellectuals. It was exhilarating.

After I failed my biochemistry midterm by not preparing for it, the fear of flunking out turned me into a disciplined student and I wound up doing much better than I had expected. During my third-year psychiatry clerkship, I was disappointed to find that it didn't really fit. The residents and the major role models I met didn't seem to be the type of person I wanted to be, whereas the residents in the internal medicine clerkship were more my type. Also, the pace of activity and the prevailing dogma in psychiatry didn't sit comfortably with me. To hedge my bets, I turned to public health as a possible alternative and did course work in tropical medicine on the side. Then after my fourth-year clerkship in psychiatry I finally concluded that the field was not for me. It was still early in my fourth year and I decided to train in internal medicine for 1 year knowing that I could go into psychiatry afterward if I changed my mind, but that didn't happen.

I never had much mechanical aptitude, so I knew that surgery was not right. I gave pediatrics some thought but I didn't enjoy the pediatric rotation. The children were suffering and often in pain, and I had to do things that made their pain worse, at least temporarily. When you're trying to get blood from a vein or to look into the ear of a crying 18-month-old child and can't explain why you're doing it, it is tough on you. Also, the constellation of illnesses in pediatrics—leukemias, developmental problems, and the like—didn't strike me as something I wanted to spend most of my life working with. As it turns out, what I saw was not a good sampling of what pediatrics is like in the real world.

When I graduated, there were no generalist fields at all. Internal medicine was all subspecialized and there was no academic family medicine anywhere in the country; there still isn't any at Harvard. A couple of my classmates wanted to be what was then called a general practitioner, and everyone tried to dissuade them. I think that one of them did go into family medicine and one went into public health.

Internal medicine was the broad part of medicine. It was more challenging and more fulfilling than I had expected. I liked the puzzling and the synthesis. Our professor of preventive medicine and public health was very bright, but I didn't see him as a role model because he didn't seem to do anything but criticize others and he never put himself on the line.

Toward the end of my first year of medical school, I tried to go back to California and engage in public health activity for the summer. However, the dean of students wanted me to do laboratory research and I wound up as a technician doing a physiologic assay in a West Coast medical school laboratory. I didn't enjoy it at all and subsequently never really considered research as a career.

Between the second and third years, I had a summer fellowship in a Boston teaching hospital that specialized in arthritis. I was on call every third night as a combination intern and laboratory technician. I did blood typing, cross-matching, and lab tests. I went on to live there my entire third year, getting room, board, and extra money. I learned a great deal about rheumatoid arthritis, but it seemed too narrow for a lifetime pursuit.

By the start of my fourth year, my interest had shifted to public health but I had no specific ideas. I thought it meant doing something for populations rather than individual patients, which tied in with my original interest in psychiatry. I felt in some unformed way that I could make a difference to thousands of patients with chronic mental health problems. Although at first I leaned toward the international aspects, as my thinking progressed I pointed my career toward trying to make a difference in the U.S. health care system.

There appeared to be only one logical option and that was internal medicine. First I would get well trained as a clinician. Then I would get into a position from which I could develop a thorough understanding of the health care system, and maybe I could try to change it. That became the simplistic reasoning behind my career plans.

I looked at internship programs on both coasts and was accepted by my fifth choice, Boston City Hospital. It was a wonderful experience. We had great residents and their teaching helped me to become a competent clinician. Because this was during the Vietnam War and doctors were being drafted, at the start of my internship I applied to the Public Health Service (PHS) to serve my military obligation. I did not support the Vietnam War.

The PHS offered two major options, the National Institutes of Health or the Centers for Disease Control (CDC)—and I got my preference, epidemiology at the CDC. After 2 years of residency, I went to Atlanta for 2 years to work on the epidemiology of enteric infections. After a 6-week course in practical epidemiology, I went on to run a national surveillance program on *Salmonella* infection. I did laboratory work on transferred antibiotic resistance in *Salmonella* (which was published), did a fair bit of speaking, and traveled around to study epidemics.

While there, I applied for a fellowship program at Harvard's Center for Community Health and Medical Care. Even though I wasn't planning on a career in internal medicine, in order to earn a credential, I decided to go for boards in internal medicine as well, and for that I needed a year in a subspecialty fellowship. So I ended up doing two fellowships simultaneously during the 2 years after CDC—one at the Harvard Center for Community Health and the other in infectious diseases at the Thorndike Lab at Boston City Hospital. I also took courses in economics, biostatistics, and advanced epidemiology. I decided against a masters in public health because I didn't want to spend time in such fields as sanitation. I figured that if I became a board-certified internist I probably would not need any more tickets. I'm not sure that I thought it all through correctly, but that's what I did.

In the fellowship, I worked on a project in which one of the Boston hospitals was trying to set up a community organization to extend health services to patients in a lower income area of Boston. I also did a lot of reading and looked for a job. By that time I had married Sally, who taught school in the Boston area. My vision of the right job for me was one that would give me responsibility for running a small, discrete medical care system where I could learn from the bottom up while doing clinical work and maybe some health services research. During my time at the CDC I had learned that writing came easily to me and I must have published about 10 papers. That was another activity I wanted to pursue.

I had a clear concept of my ideal job: half-time clinician and half-time health care administrator back in San Francisco. I tried for something with the Kaiser system there, but before they would consider me for administration they wanted me to work full time as a clinician for 3 or 4 years. If I showed leadership potential, then they would consider administrative possibilities. In the end I wound up picking the job over the place.

I joined the George Washington University Medical Center in Washington, D.C. as medical director of the outpatient clinics with responsibility for helping to start the university-sponsored health maintenance organization (HMO), of which I was to become the medical director. They took a gamble on me. I stayed for 5 years and we actually did get an HMO started. I learned a tremendous amount and made some mistakes; it was excellent training. I was meeting budgets, hiring people, designing benefits packages, looking at utilization issues, looking at the management of the outpatient system, and trying to track the use of facilities by hospitalized patients. I was also an attending on the medical service of the hospital; on the side I did unfunded health services research.

By then my wife and I had two small children and I didn't feel I was spending enough time with my family. I don't think one ever has enough time. I'd have dinner with the family and put the kids to bed, but I would get to work early and study and write during the evening hours. My wife taught school until our first child was born. She enjoyed teaching but always saw it as temporary until she became a mother. Many years later, she went back to teaching part time. She found having two small children 16 months apart stressful, but I don't think she ever felt that she had sacrificed her own career. I had the luxury of having a spouse with attitudes that were different from those of spouses of most modern physicians, men or women. It's a big, unsolved problem today.

During my years at George Washington, I got to know people in Washington, D.C. because I would go to their policy seminars and national meetings. It turned out I was in the forefront of what became a couple of national trends. One was the development of health services research and the other was the evolution of academic general internal medicine. As primary care came into its own, the Robert Wood Johnson Foundation became a big factor in its growth. As a result of my being one of the early people in what grew into a burgeoning field, I got the opportunity to consider several interesting job opportunities.

Ultimately, I was allowed to structure my own job at the University of California at San Francisco (UCSF), a once-in-a-lifetime experience. They realized that issues related to health care organization and research were going to become important to academic health centers and that it would be a good idea to have people around who could work in those areas. I guess they thought that someone like me could be useful to them. That frontier is just about closed now and the more competitive medical schools are generally pretty well stocked, but there is still a need for people in the field. I'm not sure I can say where the current frontier of medicine is because it's hard to tell, even when you're in it. One frontier might be health habits—changing individual behavior in relation to things like smoking, drug abuse, and alcoholism.

The job I designed for myself at UCSF grew out of my 5 years on the front line where I had learned a great deal about the health care system. I wanted to put some of that on paper and do research and policy analysis on the principles that lie behind health care systems—what's wrong with them and how to make them better. I wanted to do that in the Department of Medicine. UCSF had a Clinical Scholars program, an inspired hospital director, and an Institute for Health Policy Studies. I wanted to do a combination of those, to be a part-time clinician and a part-time teacher, but mainly to work on health care research as it relates to health policy. UCSF created a job that did that, and I spent 2 or 3 years at it, concerned with manpower, reimbursement, the use of health care technology, and high-cost illness. In essence, I was examining the physician as the allocator of expensive medical resources.

I felt that several things were wrong with our health care delivery system. One was the way doctors are paid. They get much too much for high technology activities and not enough for hands-on activities. I was able to develop conceptual models that made that point, and what I produced was probably the first writing in that area to point out that our medical care payment system for physicians was out of kilter.

Subsequently this has been amplified and the resource-based relative value scale that we're seeing today had its roots in some of my work. I think it's a step in the right direction, but it doesn't go far enough. The way we pay physicians ought to be neutral, and right now it isn't; there are tremendous incentives for going in some directions and against going in others. Reforming the way physicians are paid has also gotten tangled up in the whole business of the federal budget deficit. There's a movement to correct the values in the payment schedule but nothing that tries to increase the income in the underpaid specialties.

Ultimately, it's a political problem. How much should doctors make and who should decide that? What is a fair profit? Those are all political problems. Teachers are another example of underpayment by society. This nation stumbled into setting the salaries of doctors because much of the payment for medical care has become public. Until now, we have let the profession dictate what the valuation of the public payments should be, but it is increasingly appreciated that this valuation created an unfair payment system. My work contributed to that appreciation.

I was concerned also with the whole business of primary care. In Washington, I worked on health manpower needs and on reasons for academic medical centers not being sufficiently involved in primary care education. I still work on that. I did an early study, one of the first in its time, on variations in the use of resources in our own medical outpatient department. It showed that for the same kind of patients some doctors ordered tremendous numbers of laboratory tests whereas others ordered many fewer tests. That work has since been amplified by more extensive examinations of variations in medical care patterns.

I studied the epidemiology of high-cost illnesses because there was a proposed bill for catastrophic health insurance in the Congress, a bill that I thought was based on the false premise that high-cost illnesses were uncommon and concentrated in a few hospitals. I pointed out with some fairly large-scale studies that high-cost illness was a common part of the business of most hospitals and that if we created a mechanism to pay for it, we would probably do things like prolonging the life of people with terminal illness. I did a spate of studies over a 2- or 3-year period.

How things are changed politically depends on timing and circumstances. Sometimes the right study at the right time can make a difference; sometimes studies sit on the shelf for years and get snatched up when the time is right; and sometimes they may be on target but never make any difference. My work has fallen into all of those categories. You must learn not to be discouraged when your study goes on the shelf indefinitely. You must have strong interest in the field itself or you'll get frustrated.

All of the time I was doing this, I continued to be active as a clinician and teacher. It became obvious to many people at UCSF that the institution didn't have a lot of generalist capabilities. The chairman of medicine asked me to start a general medicine unit, so I spent my last 10 years there designing and staffing the unit while continuing my work in health policy analysis.

I spent about a quarter of my time seeing patients and by taking care of faculty I became something of a doctor's doctor. I regard general internal medicine as a primary care discipline and thought it was important to develop it as a field at UCSF and in the rest of the country. During my time there, I didn't see much tension between general internal medicine and family medicine, but it certainly is a generic issue. The two areas have much in common, yet academically they're often cast as rivals. We never settled it at UCSF.

I became more and more immersed in national organizations, a natural element of progressing through a career, and later on this led me to the Robert Wood Johnson Foundation. At UCSF I didn't know what I was going to do next in my career. I had the luxury of taking a sabbatical year in England where I did a comparative study of different health care systems. I looked at how different countries attack issues of manpower, use of health care technology, and care for the aged.

I came back, turned out to be a reasonably good manager, and my name began surfacing for managerial positions. One logical progression from division chief in a department of medicine is to chairman, but I decided against that. As I saw it, the modern department of medicine was dedicated to things that were not in my main experience and in which I didn't have much competence: high-technology medicine in the coronary care unit and endoscopy suite, biomolecular medicine, and research. I didn't want to direct my energies into areas where I was not particularly strong, however worthwhile they might be.

I received invitations to look at deanships, including the one at UCSF. I would have accepted it, but they didn't offer it to me. My overriding thrust was to try to make a difference in a system, and I thought that making a change in a major institution like a medical school might help. I was troubled, though, because I saw the degrees of freedom available to deans as quite limited. Still, I loved UCSF and San Francisco so much that I would have taken the job there. When I looked at other deanships, I became uncertain about what I wanted to do. Then this ideal job came up.

I don't know exactly how it came about. My job is president of the Robert Wood Johnson Foundation, which, as the nation's largest health care philanthropy, has the opportunity to fulfill the mission of improving the health and health care of this country's citizens. This is what I started out to do, and the burden is on me to make good in the arena of my choice.

I believe that what management skills I bring to the job reflect a combination of innate capacity and experience. When I was a shoe salesman and a dormitory sponsor during college, I may have exhibited some skills even then. I learned a lot in my HMO job at George Washington. I read management texts and studied people who were good managers and bad managers. I never considered getting an MBA; that's a more recent training pathway. I also got to understand myself much better. As I grew more comfortable with who I was, I became a better manager. Trying to be someone you are not doesn't work well.

For me there's probably one more job after this one, but I don't know what it will be. In an organization like this the president shouldn't stay for more than about a decade, and by then I'll be 61 and not ready to retire. I could go back to an academic setting and become a policy analyst, advisor, or consultant, or go to Washington and do something in government. My deaning opportunities have come and gone.

I try to keep a hand in seeing patients. One half-day a week I go to the local medical school where I have a panel of outpatients in the medical clinic. It's not ideal because I'm not as accessible as I want to be, but they have a group practice and colleagues there are willing to cover for me. I will try it for a year and see how it works out. My two goals for this place are to generate the best possible programs that help the country to come to grips with its pressing problems and to make it the best possible place in which to work.

As I have watched colleagues develop their careers, it has occurred to me that one mistake is to say to yourself, "I want to have a certain kind of job and I want to have it at a certain time. I'm going to set my course for that and do all I can to make it happen." You don't know what is going to happen and you don't know what you are going to be like. My advice is to do the best you can where you are and have confidence that good work will be recognized and will be its own reward. Take the time and the trouble to do your work well. Medicine offers many career opportunities, but there is tremendous gratification to be gained from the basics of medicine. The satisfaction from being able to relieve suffering, improve health, and make a difference is so ingrained in the profession that it is almost its own compensation.

Also, become comfortable with yourself by exploring your strengths and weaknesses. Learn how to capitalize on your strengths and assess whether your weaknesses are correctable. If they are, work on them; if they're not, pick opportunities in which they will not be a liability. So, if you're a good organizer but do not have much creativity, then surround yourself with creative people. If the opposite is true, then turn to the opposite solution. I've observed people who were their own worst enemies. They compounded their problems by getting themselves into situations they should have avoided.

Work with people whom you like and trust and who will tell you the truth. Put what you're doing in a broad perspective, try to see how the parts connect, and grasp the purpose of what you're doing without being sidetracked by the petty harassments and minor details that always crop up. Some people call that vision.

Have a good time. Life is short and work is a tremendous part of it. I think it was Freud who said that the two major tasks of life are work and love. You ought to love your work, if possible, and you ought to have a good time doing it. It's important to keep a sense of humor about yourself and about what you're doing. Every kind of work has its frustrations. I look back on my years and feel I've been incredibly lucky. Although they didn't necessarily seem so at the time, most of the choices I made were in retrospect logical and I feel fortunate with the way things have worked out.

To get into medical school, you must be disciplined, follow the rules, get the right grade point average and MCAT scores, and do the right things during summer vacations. Yet one of the markers of success in medicine is the ability to tolerate ambiguity. A little ambiguity is okay and students should not try to have everything all lined up because then sometimes you miss things. One of the wonderful aspects of a career in medicine is that although there are many different paths to choose, very often those paths interconnect.

I don't think there are wrong or right choices; there are degrees of rightness and wrongness. It's like getting married. If you can be happily married to one person, you can probably be happily married to many people, although I was lucky to have found a wife who has been very loving. Medicine has many opportunities, and medical students need to unwind a bit, float more, and have confidence that the tide is going with them.

Like everyone else, I can look back to some roads not taken. I've been able to maintain a reasonably good family life, follow politics, and stay active in sports as a spectator and a participant. I play tennis, climb mountains, and swim, and I've stayed reasonably fit. I've continued to read fairly voraciously—history, fiction, and current news. But I have not had as many close friends, particularly outside of medicine, and I have not been outdoors, particularly in the high mountains, as much as I would have liked. Those are two big regrets.

As for the power that comes with this job, power is seductive. You have to be conscious of the risks, surround yourself with people who will tell you the truth, and not take yourself too seriously. You must have a family that sees you as who you are and doesn't confuse you with your office. I'm sure that I will fall under the spell to some extent. But if you don't use the power, then you're neglecting one of the main tools that go with the position. Like most of life, it's a balancing act and I hope I don't get it too far off center.

Part Two

GENERALIST OR SPECIALIST

Waiting in the wings after you have chosen among the five major directions represented in the previous section is the question of whether to become a generalist or a specialist. To a great extent this decision comes down to trying to maintain a broad range of skills within a major category of medicine or narrowing your focus on a circumscribed segment of a discipline. Right now the country is taking a hard look at health personnel needs and there is great concern about the shortage of first-line, primary care physicians. Governmental inducements and pressures are being devised to draw medical school graduates toward primary care and away from specialization.

Although the external pressures cannot be ignored, you ought to resist letting them entirely overshadow your personal considerations. What kind of a life does either direction imply? In what ways will a career as a specialist or a generalist influence you as a person, as a family member, and as a doctor? How will either path mesh with your personality and aspirations?

Generalists and specialists come in different forms and shapes. Within medicine the nature of a generalist's work may be determined by the age and social context of the patients to be seen: family practice (Dr. Gould), general internal medicine (Dr. Girard), and general pediatrics (Dr. DeWitt), for example. The scope and character of a generalist's clinical activities may be established by the setting in which the care is given as in the case of emergency medicine (Dr. Heifetz) or caring for homeless people (Dr. Fantry). A physician may start a career as a specialist in a subfield of internal medicine—infectious disease, for example—and under the impact of a major phenomenon such as the current AIDS epidemic may end up serving as a general physician to a class of patients with a particular disease (Dr. Cheeseman). A surgeon who would really like to function as a generalist may find the pressures within today's setting for the practice of surgery so powerful that it becomes almost obligatory to become a specialist (Dr. Wertheimer). Specialists can concentrate on a disease category such as infectious disease (Dr. Cheeseman) or cancer (Dr. Liepman), on an organ system such as the eye (Dr. Harris) or the urinary tract (Dr. Menon), on a technology such as echocardiography (Dr. Pape), or on a procedural skill such as cardiac surgery (Dr. Vander Salm).

As a generalist you maintain close ties to your patients, you see them through many years of health and illness, you usually play a significant ongoing role in their lives, and consequently the demands on your time and emotions can be enormous. A commonly held view, especially among patients, is that a specialist seldom develops lasting relationships with patients and often becomes too tightly scheduled and, therefore, more preoccupied with the task at hand than with the patient behind the task. To some extent, society sees specialists as comparatively insensitive, aloof, and lacking in compassion and generalists as warmer and more caring. Like all such generalizations, the reality varies with the individual situation. Some specialists do, indeed, only see their patients for brief and limited encounters, whereas others become in effect the patient's primary care physician. It all depends on the nature of the illness, the needs of the patient, the personality of the physician, and the context in which the care is being given.

As with all alternatives, there are positive and negative aspects to each direction and you must take the road best traveled by you. This section presents a variety of stories about generalists, specialists, and hybrids. It illustrates how blurred the demarcations can be. Thus, even a specialist in ophthalmology, for example, may work as a generalist, as a surgically oriented clinician, as a highly subspecialized neuroophthalmologist or retina expert, or as a technology-oriented physician such as a laser expert. A range from primary care generalist to sharply limited superspecialist may be found within almost every clinical discipline these days. Where to set your sights and how to reach your goal are among the considerations covered by the stories in this section.

Chapter 6

CARING FOR THE HOMELESS

Caring for the sick and impoverished people in society ranks as one of the more venerable and benevolent traditions of medicine. Among those physicians who feel called to serve in this capacity, some go off to foreign lands to find their destined setting. Sadly enough, the opportunities to explore one's idealism in this way within the United States have burgeoned in recent decades. Tending to the homeless people in our urban centers ranks equally with going off to distant shores. How does someone decide to pursue a career of this sort? How long can one stay with it? What is it like to practice medicine under these circumstances? These are some of the questions covered during the interview in this chapter.

Dr. Lori E. Fantry is a general internist. When this interview was done, she was a member of the Department of Medicine at Johns Hopkins University Medical School, devoting the major portion of her professional time to caring for homeless people in Baltimore, Maryland. She later transferred into the Infectious Diseases Division of Johns Hopkins Hospital to work with HIV-infected patients, and subsequently began full-time studies leading to a Master's Degree in Public Health at Johns Hopkins. When she has completed that, she hopes to return to her work with indigent, HIV-infected, and homeless patients.

Lori E. Fantry, M.D., General Internal Medicine, Academic Medical Center

I had always seen myself as a primary care general internist. I had met many faculty in inspiring specialty fields, but their work didn't divert me from the homeless. . . . Especially now that I have a child of my own, I find it difficult to cope with seeing women living in the streets with a child or two.

I grew up in Binghamton, New York, with no idea that women went into medicine, even though my mother is a public health nurse. My father is an attorney, but I thought about law only briefly. At Princeton University I met women in premed, took a science course, and decided on medical school. I ended up at the Upstate Medical Center of the State University of New York in Syracuse. The tuition was right and it was close to home. Due to the lateness of my premed decision, I had a very hectic senior year. So after college I took a year-long breather for decompression and maturation. I got a summer job as a research lab tech in a Kansas City hospital. Mostly I ended up walking dogs for experiments related to antidiuretic hormone receptors, but it was interesting to be in another part of the country.

Then I went home and taught seventh grade math and science. That was helpful later because in medicine you are always teaching, whether it's patients, residents, or students. I entered medical school with a healthy attitude. After surviving the intense work at college, I told myself that getting into medical school and becoming the best doctor in the world weren't the most important issues in life. Every student could benefit from time for that kind of thinking. During the summer between my sophomore and junior college years, I was a volunteer in a hospital pediatrics unit, and in my senior year I worked in a nursing home. I could see the contrast between the two environments in that the people in the nursing home needed much more love and attention, but almost no one gave it. I guess I like the idea of helping people who really need it. Later on, working with the homeless turned out to be similar, since not many people pay attention to these individuals either.

In my first year in medical school I met my husband-to-be. He was a year ahead of me and we were married when he finished medical school and became a gastroenterologist. Otherwise, my first two years were uneventful. During my third-year clinical clerkships, I decided on internal medicine, but I loved pediatrics because of the people who go into it. As a typical student, I thought of pursuing everything, even surgery and psychiatry. I considered family medicine, but decided that since I worried about not being able to learn all there is to know about internal medicine, family medicine would be even more overwhelming.

I saw myself only as a practicing physician and not in research or even academics. I came away from psychiatry feeling that those patients were more limited by their social problems and that as a physician I would not be able to help them very much. Now, however, working in general internal medicine, especially with the homeless, I practice psychiatry quite a bit. I never considered fields like pathology or radiology because I wanted to give direct patient care. Surgery crossed my mind briefly, but a surgeon spends too much time working on people rather than with them.

As a woman in medical school, I felt some prejudice for the first time in my life. In high school, I was the only woman on the men's tennis team and never encountered problems. Then, during the third and fourth years of medical school, I began to meet resistance in surgery and similar specialties. People would predict that I'd go into pediatrics or emergency room medicine for the regular hours. That got to me. It was the first time I was ever told I couldn't do something because I'm a woman.

Today, there still are women's and men's fields in medicine. I think there are only 15 or 20 women in urology in the whole country. Fields that require a lot of training are sometimes a problem for a female. Childbearing can't be ignored: it's difficult to be pregnant, have a small child, and train, which argues against going into surgery and its subspecialties. I chose internal medicine because it was compatible with my interests and with raising a family. In medical school I planned to take 5 years off to have children, but during my residency I realized that you can't just take 5 years off from medicine.

Not having children during residency was the right decision for me. Had I been older, that would have created a dilemma. I am no longer on a resident's impossible schedule, but I do work full time and I still end up feeling that I don't spend enough time with my child. A resident with a baby must feel a lot of guilt.

It helps to have married someone who shares responsibilities. George is on call only every sixth night and every sixth weekend. We have a wonderful woman who comes in from early morning to 6 o'clock at night, and we both try to come home at a reasonable hour. Starting anew here in Baltimore has made it easier to avoid being too distracted by extra things. I keep reminding myself that someone at home needs me as much as other people do. I find it easy to put down paper work and go home to my son, but if a patient calls up and it becomes a choice between that patient and my son, that's hard.

To backtrack a bit, when I was looking for a residency, I followed my husband to the medical school of the University of Massachusetts in Worcester. Early in my fourth year, I went there for an elective, met great people, spent most of the rest of the year there, and was accepted as a resident in internal medicine. Finding a place compatible with different careers is a problem for medical couples, so we felt fortunate.

I worked hard during residency. Though I disliked being sleep-deprived, I was finally practicing medicine and enjoying it. During the third year of residency, when you take stock of where you're going, I considered going to a school of public health to look at broader health issues. I was accepted for the master's program at Harvard, but before enrolling there I took an elective month with the Department of Family and Community Medicine.

They had a segment that required a month of working with the homeless. On my first day, the person running the elective told me that they would be getting a new position for a physician assigned full time to the homeless. I said I couldn't consider it because I was pursuing a public health program, but soon I came to realize that this was really the heart of public health and I loved it. The department had clinics at the city hospital, at shelters, and at the medical school campus, and after the month ended I continued to cover clinics a few nights a week. I decided that working with the homeless was an excellent combination of clinical practice and public health, and that I would accept the job.

I had always seen myself as a primary care general internist. I had met many faculty in inspiring specialty fields, but their work didn't divert me from the homeless. Besides, I'd had enough of clinical training for a while and wanted to get to work. In retrospect an infectious diseases fellowship might have helped. To prepare to care for the homeless, one could probably use training in internal medicine, infectious diseases, psychiatry, and public health, but then one would spend her or his whole life in training and never do anything.

When I was appointed to the full-time job, it was ill defined.

It encompassed directing the medical services for the homeless in Worcester and being the physician in their clinics. Since I was the first doctor the department hired for the position, no one had a clear idea of what they wanted me to do. They were even going to let me attend public health school part time because they thought my job would be nine-to-five. I redefined my role by going in and being on call every day for a year. I put my heart into it because I wanted to provide the best care I could—the same as other patients received. I would be their doctor, something none of them had.

We set it up so that people living in the streets could get care for chronic medical problems such as hypertension as well as for acute problems. That put Worcester ahead of its time. In some shelters we ran clinics during meal times and that's how the occupants and other people coming in to eat would get to see the clinics in operation. The physical setup was not ideal; in one shelter that housed about 30 men I had to see patients in the bathroom. At that time, we concentrated on the more acute problems such as upper respiratory tract infections.

The patients were overwhelmingly grateful. In a residency people hate having you wake them at 3 o'clock in the morning when the last thing they want is another physical exam. But when I simply talked with the homeless, they were delighted. Because many of them are dirty, scruffy, and smelly, people ignore them. Just being there and talking to them made me feel great.

As in any practice, compliance issues were a problem and we had to devise solutions. The hospitals were helpful with diagnostic procedures such as X-ray studies and other tests, and the shelter for the public inebriate program transported patients to the hospital. After my residency, I continued to see my old UMass patients in the clinic at the university's hospital on Wednesday afternoons, and it was not unusual for several of my homeless patients to be there too, waiting until I was done with my regular clinic. They would get whatever was needed that night. Walk-in tests were done right away. For more complicated tests like an ultrasound study, we would make an appointment for the next day. Getting them to come back was always a problem.

If you offer homeless people medical care in the right setting, they will take it, but many are alienated by the traditional hospital and clinic systems because they can't get through the maze and hassles of registration. Often the traditional system becomes nearly impossible for homeless people to negotiate but the ones who get their care in the shelters may receive better care than the ones who have housing and have to come to the hospital clinic. One shelter had nurses on duty from 8 A.M. to 8 P.M., and a doctor came in once a week. If patients waited long enough, they could usually see the doctor on site. In contrast, people who move from a shelter to an apartment have to make clinic appointments but may not get one because they have no insurance. For medical attention, you are almost better off staying homeless. But with the new budget cuts, in most large cities the homeless and the newly housed people are experiencing the same problems getting their medical care.

One gratifying aspect of the work in Worcester was the helpfulness of my faculty colleagues. I got telephone consults quickly and could have a patient seen when necessary. Family practice faculty members covered for me in the shelters, but I was the only full timer. After I started the job, I was on call every day for a year. I had homeless patients in two hospitals just about all the time. At first, I went in on Saturday and Sunday, but after a while I just couldn't keep that up and after the first year my department worked out an on-call system with volunteers to help me on weekends.

The decision to move to Baltimore was tough for my husband and me. While he was finishing his gastroenterology training and considering staying at UMass, he began to feel that he might be overwhelmed there because the gastroenterology department was so small. He would have been on call quite a bit and was concerned about not spending enough time with our six-month-old baby. At first I was against moving but then I agreed to look around. I wanted a position working with the homeless in some city where there was an existing base, especially one linked to a university. I cried when we left Massachusetts; but Baltimore has turned out to be wonderful.

In Worcester I was able to do a lot medically for homeless people, and, in doing so, I made them happier. Some of them enjoyed the regular contact with a person who cared about them. In Baltimore, the population is very different. Here the homeless have many problems above and beyond their medical ones, many of which I can't solve. Usually when we needed someone housed for the night in Worcester, we could arrange some way to do it. In Baltimore, we really have street people who have few benefits and their problems seem tainted by a racial overtone that I didn't experience in Worcester. Here about 80 percent of the homeless people I see are black and appear to have a greater feeling of hopelessness.

My job comes under a federal program called Health Care for the Homeless (HCH). It has more than 100 units nationwide and most of them have a physician who is also affiliated with a university. Some of the units receive additional funding from state government, charities, or volunteer organizations. Here I'm affiliated with Johns Hopkins and I am an HCH physician for about 60 percent of my time. I also direct the general internal medicine residency program. My work with homeless patients is regarded as an asset in attracting people to internal medicine.

By going to one of the shelters at night, I'm doing the same sort of outreach work I used to do in Worcester. In Baltimore, the homeless people come to a downtown clinic where we can do lab tests and X-rays and provide good examining rooms and centralized care, but we miss a lot of people who will not leave the shelters. So we also go directly to the shelters, which isn't too efficient but it's a way to bring more patients into the system.

Especially now that I have a child of my own, I find it difficult to cope with seeing women living in the streets with a child or two. The children look so vulnerable, and you know that they have no hope of ever having a normal existence. We are finding second- and third-generation homelessness, which is sad.

In Worcester, I concentrated on medical problems and even tried to fight cigarette smoking. But there was also crime among the homeless, usually at the level of possessing needles or drugs and inappropriate public behavior. All this is much worse in Baltimore. Here I'm seeing hardened criminals. It still tends to be related to addiction, but it is much more serious—shooting and even killing—and that gets scary. People ask me whether the work is dangerous, especially because I'm five feet tall and weigh 100 pounds. The only time I was ever threatened was when I was getting into my car to drive away from a shelter in Worcester. Someone hanging out in the parking lot suddenly lost control and started banging on my car, but a patient of mine grabbed him and pulled him away. I've always felt protected by the other people around me.

About 80 percent of the patients are men and about 30 percent are drug addicts. I see a higher percentage of addicts in Baltimore because I work at a clinic that has nurse practitioners who refer many HIV patients to me. I'm becoming the HIV expert for the

Baltimore homeless. During my residency I wasn't particularly interested in AIDS or HIV. However, when I started working with the homeless it cropped up more and more, so that by the time I left Worcester I was following about 50 HIV patients.

Looking at the big policy picture for the homeless, in addition to solving their social problems we must eliminate the fragmentation of medical programs. More low-income housing will help, but we also need housing for specific populations. The large mentally ill population has been neglected for years. Taking them out of institutions would have been a good idea if it had been accompanied by adequate arrangements such as community mental health centers, but not much was done. A shelter is not a good place for a mentally ill person. It houses a hodge-podge of people who don't fit in anywhere—the mentally ill, the drug abusers, the alcoholics, and the women and children who have been driven from their homes by abusive spouses. We need transitional housing for all of the homeless and special housing for groups like the mentally ill, but none of that is being developed.

Funding is a problem too, but what is being spent now on medical and social problems could be put to much better use. It's being used mainly to cope with acute problems, and that's not necessarily the best thing to do. For instance, many mothers with children are housed in motels. You can imagine how expensive that is. If we established housing projects to keep them from becoming homeless in the first place, it would be cheaper and make more sense. But I'm not for building millions of low-income housing units. That was tried in the 1960s and didn't work.

Some 20–30 percent of the homeless people are women and children for whom the issue is an economic one. There's a vicious circle: women have a terrible time trying to get jobs, but if they do get a job and if they have a child, they must pay for day care even though they may earn minimum wage. That doesn't leave enough money for food and housing. To make matters worse, when a homeless woman starts working, she loses many of the benefits she had before, such as medical care under the Aid to Families with Dependent Children program.

There are big administrative and social barriers too, such as difficulty in filling out forms. Language can be another hurdle. Many homeless people qualify for benefits but don't know how to get them. Because everything is so fragmented, a worker in one program doesn't necessarily know what those in the other programs are doing.

Whoever says the homeless people prefer it as a way of life is way off-base. I have rarely met someone who chose to be homeless. Of those who appear to want to be homeless, most are mentally ill. Also, many people refuse to live in a shelter because a shelter is potentially dangerous and might carry infectious diseases. Tuberculosis among the homeless has become a serious problem in Boston and New York, and we're trying to control it here.

In the long run, I want to continue this work. I'm not making a financial sacrifice and I could stay in it even if I were the sole support of my family. I certainly wouldn't want to switch to a job that would remove me from giving hands-on medical care. I'd like to do more teaching and some research related to the medical problems of the homeless.

I think the biggest impact of my work has been attracting other doctors to it. I don't regard this as a particularly materialistic decade in medicine, but then I work with a special group of doctors. People approach me because they are interested in these issues, so I'm probably seeing the better side of medicine. And I'm seeing a steady flow of doctors into this field. Students should remember the reasons they went into medicine and stick with them. There's a great opportunity for them out there.

Chapter 7

FAMILY PRACTICE

There are physicians who have chosen their particular career direction because they enjoy talking with people, getting to know them, and trying to help them. Some of these doctors had to overcome the negative attitudes of classmates and teachers as they headed for family practice or its congeners. Now an even greater problem seems to be stemming from contemporary changes in the nature of clinical practice—the paper work, the regulations, and the economics are all impinging on a doctor's time for talking with patients. Still, practitioners such as Dr. Gould hang in there, hoping for a turnaround of some sort.

Dr. John H. Gould practices family medicine in Falmouth, a town on Cape Cod in Massachusetts. He holds an appointment as assistant professor of family medicine at the School of Medicine of the University of Massachusetts Medical Center.

John H. Gould, M.D., Family Medicine, Private Practice

I like talking to people about their problems, getting to know them and the context of their illness, and maybe preventing some problems. . . . In academic medicine the disease sometimes becomes more important than the person, but I was always more interested in the person who was ill than in the possibility that they had some rare lupus variant. You absolutely need academic excellence, yet you also have to care about who the patient is.

I went into medicine almost by default. When I was young, I hated doctors because they gave me shots. I went off to college to study for the foreign service, but after a semester of struggling with language I decided that wasn't for me. But I also didn't want to get a job just yet, so at age 18 I enlisted in the air force for 4 years, trained as a medical lab technician, and was assigned to Otis Air Force Base on Cape Cod. Nights and weekends I moonlighted at Falmouth Hospital, a small hospital with one technician, a couple of internists, four or five general practitioners, a surgeon, and an obstetrician. I came to admire what they did for patients and as time passed people began to expect that I too would become a doctor.

After I left the service I worked for a microbiologist at the Woods Hole Oceanographic Institution and also remained employed with the hospital. Six months later I returned to college on the G.I. bill, studied microbiology, and finished in 3 years. Toward the end of college I applied to medical school. I was 25, had worked in the field, and knew where I was going. I applied mainly to East Coast medical schools and got into Harvard.

By then I knew that I wanted to become a general practitioner. It probably went back to my time at the Falmouth Hospital. When I was there, I never considered surgery. I admired some of the general surgeons but didn't like trauma because I preferred living, talking patients. I wanted to deliver babies and take care of heart attacks, diarrhea, or whatever. Besides, the thought of having to save somebody who was near death frightened me.

The other drawback was the long hours. One of the surgeons there was a wonderful person, but he seemed to be in the hospital all of the time. I didn't want to live like that. I enjoyed watching general practitioners, internists, and pediatricians talking to their patients and watching people recover and leave the hospital. I got to know patients with chronic illnesses. Seeing individuals go downhill was depressing, but I was willing to take on that side of medicine.

Nowadays the medical students who sign up for elective work in my office aren't thronging into primary care. Finance must be a big factor. Many are in heavy debt for their educational costs. I never worried about the money, but it was a lot less expensive 20 years ago. I took out loans, received some scholarship money, my parents helped, and I worked nights at the hospital blood bank. I ended up owing only about $7500, compared to the $60,000 to $100,000 average today.

Starting out now, I might think twice about going into primary care because it's tough unless you're independently wealthy. Perhaps society should take on the indebtedness of students who go into primary care or maybe just pay the primary care physicians more equitably. The other problem is that primary care specialties haven't been given very much status. At Harvard that didn't bother me because in the early 1970s you just did your own thing. My vision was to be a family doctor in some little town, and I got there.

To become a primary care physician you need inner desire, but it also has to be nurtured from the outside. To some extent this was encouraged at Harvard. A small "Family Health Care Program" took 20 students in the third year and assigned them several families to follow. I joined and was assigned to a pediatrician, a family doctor from New Hampshire, and a nurse practitioner. We had regular meetings about social issues and were on call for our patients all of the time. If I was in class and one of my patients became sick, I had to get away to see him or her. I would try to arrive at a diagnosis and then discuss it with the preceptor. The families knew I was a student but they appreciated my involvement. That was my best experience at Harvard. It is unfortunate that the chief of medicine at the Brigham abolished the program in the late 1970s.

In academic medicine the disease sometimes becomes more important than the person, but I was always more interested in the person who was ill than in the possibility that they had some rare lupus variant. You absolutely need academic excellence, yet you also have to care about who the patient is. Sometimes in my practice I go off on my own tangents, but I do my best to focus on the patient and the disease. You teach that by example. Some of my teachers were cold fish and others were great at it. Superspecialization has made the academic setting less conducive to concern for the patient as a human being, but in the end it all depends on the individual doctor.

When I was taking a cardiology elective at the Brigham, one of the instructors appeared to feel that a patient's heart was the most important facet of care and that it was almost a mechanical pump. But then there was Dr. Dexter, a famous cardiologist who impressed me one day when we were making rounds. We saw an old man whose abdominal aortic aneurysm had been repaired and who had suffered a little postoperative confusion. He was concerned that he might have said some inappropriate things. As we were all leaving the room, Dr. Dexter went back, leaned over, and said, "When I had mine fixed, I did the same thing." The man smiled, thanked Dr. Dexter, and shook his hand. That was the mark of a humane physician.

The specialist should try not to be solely a supertechnician. When I refer patients to a specialist, they're scared and have many questions, but they hesitate to bother the new doctor because he looks too busy. I don't know why that happens. Too often, specialists seem to want to get a procedure done and don't spend enough time with the patient. Even I have done that when pressured. But if I feel that I did not give the patient in the office the time he or she needed, I make up for it on the next visit. Spending time with patients is what I like, but it's not right for everybody. Some doctors really should be mainly technicians.

When as a first-year medical student I made it known that I intended to go into primary care, my classmates and teachers tried to argue me out of it. What strengthened my resolve was the fact that somebody there was doing it. Had I gone to a medical school without a family practice department, as is now the case at Harvard, it would have been much more difficult. Role models make a difference in favor of a field—or against it. I learned that when I spent the summer before medical school taking a course at the Marine Biological Laboratory in Woods Hole. Even though there were Nobel laureates all over the place and it was fun working among them, I realized that I didn't want to do it for the rest of my life.

I never considered psychiatry because I wanted more variety and because sometimes I had trouble telling the psychiatry residents from the patients. I liked pediatrics, but I wanted contact with older people too. Internal medicine by itself wasn't enough either— mainly older people with chronic illnesses. To do the same thing day after day, like taking out cataracts or replacing heart valves, though challenging, seemed repetitious and boring. I like talking to people about their problems, getting to know them and the context of their illness, and possibly preventing problems. Many other branches of medicine involve fixing but not preventing.

During the obstetrics part of my residency, I found that I did not like delivering babies and doing C sections. It was mostly hours of boredom interrupted by moments of terror. Even so, I liked caring for newborns.

By the beginning of the fourth year, I was committed to a residency in family practice. It had become a recognized specialty and there wasn't much primary care in internal medicine at the time. Even if there had been, I still would have picked family practice because of the pediatrics. Early in the fourth year, I spent a 1-month elective with a family doctor in Gardner, Massachusetts. Seeing how hard he worked gave me pause, but I finally decided that even though I couldn't work as hard as he, I could still enter his field.

It concerned me that I might end up only partially trained in several fields whereas I wanted to be thought of as expert in everything. Yet pediatric nurse practitioners are capable of doing most of what pediatricians do. Indeed, you need pediatricians for perhaps 10 percent of what's done for kids, and the same holds true for internists and adult patients. By and large, it's for the 10 percent that we really need the pediatricians and the internists, and I can always call in one of them for cases I can't manage. I'm not afraid to ask for help and knowing when to do that is an important part of my work. I always want the best for my patients and there's no shame in seeking another opinion.

A primary care physician can set limits on his or her schedule by not doing obstetrics, by not seeing patients in the ICU, or by not doing procedures such as sigmoidoscopies in the office. To set those limits, you need an adequate specialty backup in the community, so that in a rural area you must learn to do those things for yourself. I'm comfortable with what I do here. There's always been a lot of backup help. We have four cardiologists, two gastroenterologists, and a few neurologists. I liked dermatology because it's noninvasive, so I learned a little on my own. I'm no great dermatologist, but I know a little bit more than the average family physician. My motivation was personal because I have had psoriasis since I was 19. A chronic problem like that has made a difference in my approach to my patients, especially those with skin problems.

There were no family practice residencies in Massachusetts when I applied and there were only about 10 in the whole country. Family medicine had become a recognized specialty in 1969 and I started training in 1974. I chose Rochester because I learned a lot about the place during the day I spent there for interviews and I came away feeling that it was good and that it was right for me.

The outpatient part of the residency turned out to be extremely helpful for learning about the reasons behind medical problems. When someone came in with a complaint, why did they come that day? The challenge was to learn the story behind the story. Every visit was potentially amazing. People would come in with a sore throat and within 5 minutes be telling you about the real trouble at home. It was incredible, if you took the time to listen. As a resident I felt I had all the time in the world to give to my patients. I was being paid a salary and didn't have to worry about money. I still derive extraordinary gratification from my interactions with patients, but it is tempered by lack of time. I feel pressure to make it from payroll to payroll in the office.

After the 3 required residency years, I was free to go out and practice, and it was a strange feeling. Since leaving the service in 1967, I'd been working to become a doctor. Ten years later, the train pulled into the station and I got off, not at all sure about anything and wondering what to do next. Everybody else was married, had kids, and knew what they were going to do. I hadn't planned ahead. I applied to the National Health Service Corps but to this day haven't heard from them.

After residency I took a couple of months off with friends on Cape Cod. There I met someone in the Family Practice Department at Hershey Medical School who invited me to visit their residency program in Altoona, Pennsylvania. They had two American and three Pakistani residents, and all their faculty had quit. They offered me the job of directing the residency program. It seemed like an interesting challenge, so I accepted. I did administrative work, taught, and saw my own patients several half days a week, but, as always, there were hassles. After 4 years I quit and came back here. When I left, there were 18 American residents, and I was proud of having built up the program.

I took a few months off and met a general internist looking for someone to cover his practice while he went on a summer sabbatical. When he came back he invited me to stay on. We practiced together for 5 years and then he decided to leave medicine. I went on my own 4 years ago.

My work day starts with morning rounds in the hospital, where I have one to ten patients. Then I check X-rays, do paper work, or meet with a hospital committee. Someone sick may call and I will see them in the emergency room and admit them if necessary. I usually get to the office around 10 A.M., where I take half an hour to return phone calls and then see patients. I may see six people in the morning. From noon to 1 P.M., I do mail and paper work, taking 15 minutes to eat a sandwich. I see patients again from 1 until about 5 P.M., and then I go back to the hospital. I'm on call about every third night. Four of us cover for each other.

I see patients in all age groups. Being in family practice allows me to relate to them over a long time. I've known some of them for 9 years and sometimes when they come in I can sense what's wrong. I know their stresses and I know their families. I enjoy being part of their lives, but to spend enough time with them I've had to learn to work faster.

I've been the school physician for the town of Bourne since I came here. Medical students work in my office for a 1-month elective about three or four times a year. I enjoy watching them become excited about patients and their problems, and they get a chance to see what happens in real life.

I got married 7 years ago and have a 16-year-old stepson. Even though I try to make enough time for my family, I often miss out on things. For instance, my son is in the school band and so far I've been on call during each of their concerts. Sometimes I have second thoughts about my career and wish I had a job that involved 40 hours a week. I'm considering joining a health maintenance organization, but I like the freedom here and so I'm ambivalent about it. I guess I can't have it both ways.

I'm interested in computers and in making information available faster to practicing physicians. At the hospital I'm working on hooking up their new computer system so that in addition to entering orders and diets, we can also get X-ray and lab reports on the patient floor. The computer in my office is primarily for practice management—billing and other forms, the biggest information burden. I can also search through patient diagnoses and visits and print letters asking people to come in for a flu shot or a mammogram.

I don't think I'll stay in practice until I'm 90. Eventually I might want to do something else. My patients are like family, though, and

I don't want to leave them, even when they call at 5 o'clock in the morning. It would be nice to work more efficiently, and I'd like the patients to be more involved in their own care.

I see nursing home patients, and they take a lot of my time. Because I want to cut back on my work hours, I'm allowing the number to fall off by attrition. What I don't know is who will take care of the elderly in the future. That's a big problem and somehow geriatrics has got to be made more attractive as a field. Sixty percent of my time is devoted to the elderly here.

I've grown personally in the years since I finished my training, but I've also regressed. I used to read more. I loved poetry in college and was hungry to learn all sorts of things. I devoured arts and literature but have no time for that now. It would be great to simply go jogging, but when I tried it I'd soon get beeped and have to go back.

It seems to me that a couple of decades ago doctors were more interested in and enthusiastic about going into family practice than they are now. Part of it may be the fault of the specialty but part of it is due to the changes in medicine. With all of the federal and state regulations, I feel like an employee of Medicare with little room for my own initiative. When you admit somebody to the hospital, you have to make sure that the patient meets the criteria of this or that committee and review board. Someone is always lurking in the background, like a buzzard sitting on your shoulder and looking down. If you order a CAT scan it may be rejected for payment after the fact.

Nevertheless, there will always be a need for the core things that a physician does: taking a history, doing a physical, deciding what might be wrong with the patient, and determining which way to go. One big question is how many tests to do. There's the unspoken fear of being sued for malpractice, and I do practice defensive medicine. If you don't, you're foolish. Although I do more tests now than I did at first, it may not be all bad. Sometimes the extra tests surprise you and reveal something important. Years ago, when we were trying to do without tests in family practice, we tended to pass too many things off as psychosomatic. A patient can have all kinds of stress, and the problems that stress creates, and also have a brain tumor. So I try to parallel the two approaches.

With all of the changes in family practice, the relationship with patients is still the best part, but there are hassles even with them.

The biggest hassle is when they expect me to know all about their Medicare benefit form. After I save their life, they get mad because Medicare didn't cover it. Medicare and the insurance companies ought to educate patients about their insurance policies instead of leaving it to us. The patients feel that because they've paid for the insurance they're covered and it's up to the doctor to take care of it. The insurance companies have to take responsibility and not pass the burden to us.

Maybe a one-payer system would be simpler and eliminate some administrative details. If I could see my patients and not have to make sure I get the right code entered or worry about why this or that was rejected, the practice of medicine would be much better. I have to do all that because I've been turned into a businessman and I'd rather not be a businessman. I went into family practice with idealistic motives that are becoming undermined by the system in which I have to work.

Now and then I fumble toward something like socialized medicine, but that has its problems too. I saw it in military medicine, where patients were pieces of meat at the whim of the system. At least in private practice the doctor has to meet the patients' expectations or they'll leave.

The answer probably involves a mixture of steps. What I want is to alleviate the economic pressure enough to enable me to spend more time with my patients. Pay me more for the time I spend so I can cover my overhead. Primary care doctors are not reimbursed for the time they spend with Medicare patients.

In the future, medical practice is going to become more regulated and even more irritating. Even though I feel this way, I can still be an encouraging mentor to medical students. After all, they're already in medicine. I try to give them a realistic view and help them see both sides. If my son wanted to go into medicine, I would certainly support his decision, but he ought to know what it's like and take special pains to make time for his family and personal interests.

My parting message for the students who will read this is that you have to find the part of medicine that meets your inner needs. If you're happy working 18-hour days, then become a surgeon. If you like going home at 5 to play with your kids, then find some other specialty. I think finding time with your family is probably the bottom line. Match that up with your other needs and look around to see who's achieving that. Maybe it means being an ophthalmologist or a dermatologist and they can do superb work from 10 to 5.

To be prepared to make this decision in the third or fourth year of medical school, you must pay careful attention during the different clinical rotations. Students who spend time here get a feeling for what my life is like. Another helpful part of it comes from the impression faculty members make on you, but it's important to see past their mentor role. You may really like the way Dr. Z practices medicine, but you've also got to imagine what things are like when he gets home at night.

Sit down with fellow students and talk about how one goes about choosing. This book will make a good beginning for talking. Bring in doctors from the community and ask, "If you were starting now, what would you do differently?" In the end, though, you'll decide for yourself and you'll do it with your heart and not your head.

Chapter 8

EMERGENCY MEDICINE

Emergency medicine is a maturing branch of medicine that has come into its own during the past decade or two as the patterns by which medical care is delivered have changed dramatically. In some ways emergency medicine represents a distillation of the essential elements of a wide range of specialties since, as Dr. Heifetz points out, the emergency room (ER) physician aspires to expertise in the management of the acute phase of the diseases seen by specialists in virtually all fields of medicine. In other ways emergency medicine lacks key attributes and gratifications of other clinical disciplines in that the ER physician is rarely afforded an opportunity to develop long-term ties to a patient. In any event, according to Dr. Heifetz, "emergency medicine is here to stay."

Dr. Irvin N. Heifetz is the clinical director of the Emergency Department of the hospital at the University of Massachusetts Medical Center in Worcester and an assistant professor of medicine in its school of medicine.

Irvin N. Heifetz, M.D., Emergency Medicine, Academic Medical Center

The patients don't want to spend a lot of time with you, and you don't have a lot of time to devote to them, so you must quickly establish relationships of mutual trust. I have to

trust them to tell me what's really bothering them and they
have to trust me to listen and to make my best decision. . . .

My mother taught school and we lived above my father's dry cleaning store in Lawrence, Massachusetts. Medicine was not my childhood dream. I first thought about it in college. My parents didn't push me into it, but they're happy that I'm in it. My dad is an amateur singer and I guess I inherited some of his talent. In school I sang in occasional musical productions and considered a career in music. As a matter of fact, I still do.

In high school, at Phillips Academy, I most enjoyed language and literature. I was not much of a scientist but I was curious about how thing work. When I went on to the University of Massachusetts in Amherst, I realized that to be well educated one ought to know some science and math.

At first I considered writing or teaching for a career, and then it dawned on me that somehow I had fulfilled the premedical requirements. I felt that I was unlikely to write the great American novel and that medicine was interesting and a good way to try to help people. Because becoming a doctor required 4 more years of schooling followed by 3 to 5 years of training, I took a break after college and taught high school for a year. Then I entered the medical school of the University of Massachusetts, here in Worcester.

I started with no inclination toward a specific area. Early on, I considered psychiatry because it relates to language and therefore to my interest in writing. Eventually, I chose internal medicine—but it was a close call. I had become more interested in the biological aspects of life and was influenced by the people I met in internal medicine. I was encouraged to apply for a medicine residency in Worcester, and I stayed for 3 more years.

Although I'm still not sure whether I might not have enjoyed psychiatry more, another reason I didn't go into it was that back then the department was not very good. It's hard to know whether I have regrets. In general, what you are today is the result of all your prior experiences and I'm reasonably happy with what I am now. Had I gone the other route, I might have been a different person and, perhaps, less pleased with myself.

I remember thinking seriously about surgery. In fact, I regret not having more surgical skills. In ER work, you do many minor surgical procedures as well as major procedures for trauma stabilization, and

I enjoy them. Surgery was not appealing in medical school, partly because my clerkship rotation was not great and partly because I didn't want to spend 5 hard years in training and then 35 long years practicing general surgery.

In the pediatric rotation we had very good faculty but we spent all our time on the inpatient service where we saw mainly the unfortunate graduates of the Neonatal Intensive Care Unit. They were not disasters but neither did they do all that well. I knew there were other, more encouraging kinds of problems in the pediatric world at large but they weren't there on the fifth floor.

I saw myself as a general primary care internist and not as a subspecialist. I spent my first medical school summer working with a cardiologist. He didn't draw me into his specialty, but he did help me to decide that I would be happy seeing patients. Throughout my residency, I spent time at the Tri-River Clinic, a primary care facility associated with this medical school, where I met a couple of internists worth emulating. I settled even more firmly into the path that would lead to their kind of practice. Midway through my last year of residency, I considered going to Tri-River, staying at Worcester in the primary care clinic, or joining a group practicing in Andover.

Then, out of the blue, I was invited to join a friend who had just started to run a community hospital ER 40 miles west of here. He had completed 3 years in internal medicine and a year here in emergency medicine. He recruited me and several of my medicine colleagues, and out we went. In addition, I accepted a second, part-time appointment here in the ER.

This arrangement was a major shift from internal medicine, but I wasn't thinking about long-term implications. I just felt that I was fairly good at ER work, whatever that was, and I did not regard my decision as a permanent move but rather as a good first step away from "Mother" UMass. Besides, except for the major trauma, the sickest ER patients have emergencies involving internal medicine—heart attacks, diabetic coma, the pneumonias, and the arrhythmias.

Most of my colleagues in emergency medicine, especially those who trained specifically for the field, regard it as a surgically oriented way of life, but I don't. Certainly, surgical work comes into play, as do things an internist is not trained for but which the mythical, complete emergency medicine physician should be able to do. You encounter sprains, fractures, and lacerations; fevers in children;

some dermatologic disorders; and this and that. One can't do everything, but the variety is attractive, and my choice wasn't altogether by default. Faced with my uncertainty about joining a medical practice, I was attracted to the idea of spending a year in the ER, making a few bucks and having some time off.

What bothered me then, and still does, was the lack of full patient interaction. What the ER demands, perhaps more than any other setting, is the ability to establish instant rapport with patients. Contrary to general impression, in ER work, even at facilities that treat many patients with head injury, we work mostly with conscious patients. The patients don't want to spend a lot of time with you, and you don't have a lot of time to devote to them, so you must quickly establish relationships of mutual trust. I have to trust them to tell me what's really bothering them and they have to trust me to listen and to make my best decision, even though I may have an ear cocked to the monitor on the arrhythmia patient in the next bed. It's a distinctive skill.

The more efficient we are, the sooner our patients move on, and so we don't often get to see the outcome of a problem. That isn't too fulfilling. Some patients use the ER for their primary care—I have a few dozen—and they generate relationships similar to those of an internal medicine practice. But it's not the same and I miss long-term associations where you're the "real" doctor.

As a board-certified specialty, emergency medicine is only about 15 years old. I was certified by "grandfathering" (qualifying to take the Board examination on the basis of 5 years of clinical experience instead of a formal residency) and did not take another residency, but there are jobs now advertised for which I would not qualify because they require emergency medicine training. Yet I am happy to have acquired some capabilities which that training does not provide. An emergency medicine residency includes 4 months in internal medicine, a month or two in intensive care or coronary care, and equivalent time in the surgical intensive care unit (ICU), on the trauma service, in orthopedics, and, perhaps, in ophthalmology. Residents do a few months of pediatrics, a month or two of obstetrics, and about 12 months in the ER. But none of my ER colleagues has the foggiest idea, except perhaps from personal or family experience, what it's like for a patient to have a chronic illness or what it's like to be that patient's doctor. It is in clinic experience that you learn to appreciate how emergency medicine should go beyond just making a diagnosis, stabilizing the situation, and getting the patient out.

At times an ER can be a 30-ring circus. Some days most of my energy is directed to finding a bed; getting someone off telemetry so the next patient can get on it; begging, borrowing, and sometimes stealing the last ICU slot for a patient already in the ER rather than for someone who is on the way in; or tracking down a consultant to see a patient, not so much because I don't know what to do but to help the consultation services to train their residents and fellows.

I'd like to think I do well at bringing humaneness to the job, but at times I go home wondering whether I missed something that was worrying a patient because I had to move briskly, or because it was one long, rotten day and I just didn't quite have enough heart left at 3 A.M., or because some of the cynicism that exists in emergency medicine, as it does in other fields, has rubbed off on me. I'm talking about the cynicism of "Here comes another drunk" or "Here comes another IV drug abuser" or "Here comes another cranky old lady" or "Here comes another patient with a hang nail, waking me up at 3 in the morning." I put these in what I hope are the quotes of others, although on occasion I'm guilty of those feelings myself.

To wrap it up, in emergency medicine we treat acute problems. We provide the initial medical care and then work the system to move the patient to the right next place—be it the hospital bed, the clinic, or the patient's home for continuing care. We see patients of all ages, from babies on up. We try to create a humane interaction during our involvement, but often we don't get to see what happens to the patient. We are often called "jacks of all trades and masters of none." But that is not true. We strive to master the acute aspects of virtually all of the other specialties. Emergency medicine is not age-defined as are pediatrics and geriatrics, not organ-defined as are cardiology and gastroenterology, and not disease-defined as are oncology and infectious disease. It's really time-defined in hours.

You have to be the doctor who knows as well as or better than the neurologist how to manage acute seizures. Most neurologists don't see people seizing; they see them later. Most cardiologists don't see people having myocardial infarctions or arrhythmias; they see them later in the ICU. Most general surgeons are not the first ones to see an acute abdomen; rather, it's someone in the ER or the private or clinic office. What it is like in the ER depends a lot on where you are. For example, here we have a helicopter that brings in many trauma patients.

I have irregular hours, and the stress can be pretty high, but I can't say whether it exceeds that of a family practice physician in a demanding community. Each doctor probably thinks that his or her field is the most stressful. One sick patient with an unstable myocardial infarct or unstable trauma can be worrisome, but in the ER you never have just one patient and you rarely have just one very sick one.

When I worked at the community hospital, I had no administrative responsibility. When I was on I worked for 12 hours and occasionally for 24; but when I was off nobody called me. On average an ER physician works 36–48 hours a week, and people share the good and the bad hours. The older I get (I'm 40), the longer it takes me to bounce back from night shifts but now I work only two or three of them a month.

In my off hours I sing in a chorus and take music lessons. I'm in an opera workshop this semester. I'm not married yet. As for my professional growth, I've become pretty good at things I didn't learn in medical school or residency. I haven't published much or risen far in the academic hierarchy. I am a clinical director, which I'm happy to be. I don't anticipate a change in the foreseeable future. During the last few years I have had invitations to become ER director in private community hospitals or in other hospitals affiliated with academic health centers, but I have elected to stay here.

My teaching is mainly at the bedside. Virtually every patient who comes to the ER is seen by an intern or a resident, and I see the patients with them. Medical students rotate through the department for a week as part of their internal medicine clerkship, and we offer a popular 1-month elective in the fourth year. I give only a few formal didactic lectures per year.

Emergency medicine has changed during my 10 years. It's better accepted, but as a new hybrid specialty it lacks the cachet of surgery, medicine, or the other well-established subspecialties. With the recent decline in the popularity of internal medicine and with the decline, perhaps, in the quality of people going into internal medicine, our residents have been outstanding in comparison.

The shift of choice from internal medicine to ER medicine is related to the frustrations with such things as diagnostic-related groups (DRGs), third-party overseers, and conflicting or counterproductive government regulations. You are relatively protected from that stuff in the ER where most doctors are on a salary, which they receive whether they see 100 patients in a day or 10, and where malpractice insurance and health and disability coverage are all taken care of.

Emergency medicine is here to stay. As medical care has tended to concentrate in the outpatient setting, people have tended to use the ER more. People who may have been sent home prematurely often come back with a problem not as well resolved as it might have been had the rules permitted another day or two in the hospital. There will always have to be at least one ER in any major population area, a place to go any day or night for any kind of medical problem. Perhaps only 15 percent of the patients seen in the ER have a problem that truly could not have waited until the next day, but many people don't have physicians, many don't have insurance, and some just don't understand the proper role of their doctor versus the ER.

I don't know what I'll be doing 20 years from now, but if I were ever to decide to make a career change, my boards in internal medicine plus some retooling would make me fairly salable. If current trends continue I will be in great demand in internal medicine, but I don't know whether I would want to do it. Although I could go back to being an internist, most of the people who train in emergency medicine today could not. However, they do have other alternatives. Many toxicologists come from emergency medicine, and occupational medicine and administration also come to mind. Then again, if I decided to leave medicine entirely, Broadway might beckon.

I would recommend my career to students, but I would recommend internal medicine too. Students should enter with as much advance knowledge as possible. You can't really know a field until you work in it, but that's an expensive way to learn anything. By reading articles and books like this one, by talking to people, and by learning about yourself, you have to fit yourself to your job as well as you can. If you can match your personality with the personality of the field, then you've got something good. If it's a mismatch, then you've got a problem. Fortunately, you can often find out early on and switch.

Chapter 9

GENERAL INTERNAL MEDICINE

If he hadn't enrolled in a program of the U.S. Public Health Service to cover his medical education costs, in all likelihood Dr. Muller would never have settled in Uxbridge, Massachusetts as a general internist in what was at first a medically underserved community. Certainly, the community has benefitted from his career decision; it is comforting to know that Dr. Muller feels that he has too.

Dr. William G. Muller is a general internist who works for the University of Massachusetts Medical Center in a satellite health care clinic in Uxbridge, Massachusetts. He is an associate professor of medicine in the Department of Medicine of the medical school. In addition to his administrative work, he cares for patients and teaches medical students and residents.

William G. Muller, M.D., General Internal Medicine, Community Health Center

The best thing about what I do is getting to know people over a long time line and providing continuity of care. . . . It seems that people going into a subspecialty must feel somewhat overwhelmed by the totality of medicine and that they choose to master just some of it and leave the rest to others. A primary care physician tries to master most of it, and the biggest challenge is to know when you're in over your head.

My home town is Andover, Massachusetts. My parents were from working class backgrounds. In high school I was oriented toward science, not art, music, or business. I think I was influenced to choose medicine mostly because my biology teacher had come to regret his own decision not to become a doctor. From high school I went to Harvard College as a premed.

My one regret about college is not branching out more. I took courses in nineteenth and twentieth century art and wrote long papers about such matters, but I wish I had done more with music, for example. When I was accepted into the "society of educated men," I should have been required to be broader in my training.

I survived organic chemistry and went to medical school in Vermont. Although it was not a research-oriented institution and it prepared students almost exclusively for the practice of medicine, I had to go there no matter how I felt about practice or research because it was the only school I got into. Another factor was cost. The University of Massachusetts medical school was in its infancy and the state had a contractual agreement with the University of Vermont to admit students there at the in-state tuition level of $950 a year.

My most significant mentor was an invasive cardiologist who had trained at Johns Hopkins, planning initially to be a surgeon. I met him when I was a sophomore, and he provided the counsel and letters of recommendation I needed to find a residency. I tried to go through my clinical rotations without preconceived notions, unlike some of my classmates who knew, perhaps from birth, that they wanted to be surgeons.

When I was a sophomore medical student, I joined the Public Health Service (PHS) Scholarship Program because I was concerned about incurring too large an educational debt. By current standards that sounds absolutely insane because I was worried about an eventual total debt of about $20,000. Today the average debt is about $100,000—a major determinant in choosing a career in medicine, and one that needs corrective action.

I was oriented to being a practitioner, in part because that was the basic thrust of my medical school. I had one summer free in medical school and worked on a project where we identified families who had been chronic visitors to the emergency room, had multiple problems, and so on. We tried to improve their utilization of the health care system and their life circumstances in general. I learned more about interacting with patients from that experience than I had in the first year of medical school.

I met my cardiologist mentor in a course for integrating clinical subjects with the basic sciences. He was an attending when I was on cardiology and I maintained close contact with him throughout medical school. Cardiology is my favorite subspecialty in medicine, and I would have gone into it if I had continued in subspecialty training. Instead, I signed up with the PHS in my second year. They paid for my schooling and gave me a stipend. In return, I agreed that after my residency training I would practice, 1 year for each year of support, in what they designated as a medically underserved area. This was the beginning of the PHS Scholarship Program.

There was an element of wanting to save the world among those of us who signed up. As children of the 1960s, we were a fairly altruistic crew. We sensed that something was wrong and felt that we didn't have to let things remain the way they had been for decades. Although money was relevant to my decision to join the PHS, no one indentures himself without some other motivation. Service in the armed services would have paid better, for example, but I wasn't interested.

In addition to financial help, the PHS offered one a chance to train where one wanted, to stay in the competitive marketplace, to go into the program that one was most qualified for, to practice in a structured situation, and to work in an underserved area. It was altruism without much personal compromise. It gave me 3 years to try out practice before making a lifetime commitment. Students and residents are asked to make decisions prematurely in their training. Incentives should be developed for people to leave their track for a time to see whether primary care practice would be to their liking. I suspect what happened to me would happen to others. They would find that they liked it and didn't need to do angioplasty procedures and so forth to derive professional satisfaction.

I chose to enter an internal medicine residency. I did consider other primary care specialties such as family practice and pediatrics. I went through each clinical rotation trying to envision myself in that field. I never saw myself in psychiatry; it was too touchy-feely and not sufficiently based in the biological sciences. I did surgery in January in Vermont and had to start rounds at 5:30 in the morning when it was about 30° below outside. Any inclination toward sur-

gery was stifled in that rotation. I saw medicine as being the least
limiting.

Today, when students ask for my advice about family practice, I
tell them two things. First, think about where you are planning
to practice. In an urban state like Massachusetts, family practice
physicians have difficulty defining their niche. Although some family practice training programs teach surgery and obstetrics, most
hospitals in Massachusetts are not likely to allow a family practice
doctor to do either. But in other places, northern New England particularly, they need family practice people who will do surgery and
obstetrics. The training that internists get is not appropriate for that
kind of setting. A student ought to visit family practitioners in the
area where he or she wants to settle, see what they do there, and get
their views on the kind of training that would constitute the best
preparation.

Second, evaluate how sure you are about what you want to do. If
you are absolutely sure, fine; but many students are not. Some may
decide later that they like cardiology and then have to backtrack
into an internal medicine program. It can be done, but not easily.
Family practice has done a better job of training people to work in
primary care than internal medicine has. Internal medicine started
primary care training in reaction to losing students to family medicine but they used subspecialty-trained physicians to do the teaching. Only people in primary care know what a primary care doctor
is, so they ought to do the training.

For my own residency, I went to the University of Wisconsin, a
subspecialty-oriented center. I wanted to train in a university program, but having come to like Vermont I did not want to go back to
a major metropolitan area. I wasn't leaving the Northeast indefinitely; I always planned to return. I had been married a couple of
days after graduation from college to a woman who, like me, was
from Andover.

Wisconsin was a melting pot and the school had a very good
program. I discovered that the criteria for choosing a residency program should include factors like who your fellow residents are because you learn as much from them as you do from attendings.
Wisconsin had a large VA hospital where the house staff controlled
almost everything, they had good community hospitals, and they
were involved in primary care.

As my residency came to an end and the time was near for deciding where the PHS would send me, my anxiety mounted because I suddenly realized that they owned me and could send me anywhere. The choice of region was not my own. What was worse, there were more people who wanted to go to New England than could be accommodated.

The selection of locations to qualify as practice sites was based on federal legislation that decreed whether a place was a Health Manpower Shortage Area. The most common arrangement in a practice site was that a local community board would build or lease a building and the corps would provide the physician manpower. There was community control in a partnership with the federal government. The physician would work for the federal government and report to the community board.

I interviewed in several places and saw various arrangements. In some places you were just talking to several prominent people in a community with a hospital situated 50 miles away and they wanted you merely to run an outpatient clinic. I recall interviewing in a rural town in Maine where the nearest hospital is the Maine Medical Center in Portland, 45 miles away. The setting, the foothills of the White Mountains, was in the peak of the foliage season. It was fantastic, but they expected me to do pediatrics and I hadn't been trained in it. Trainees in family practice were best suited for that sort of environment.

I remember an arrangement in upstate New York, which required working with small communities around Cortland, near Syracuse. They had three outlying clinics surrounding a central community hospital and staffed by physician assistants. The doctor went to one clinic one day, another clinic the next day, and was a circuit rider who provided hospital care for the clinic patients. It was an opportunity for creative thinking about how to deliver health care services in sparsely populated areas.

I also interviewed in Dexter, Maine, the shoe town. They had a small, wood frame hospital with about 10 beds. During the interview they said they had authorization to give blood transfusions, and, indeed, they had done one about 3 years ago. In contrast, a community up the road had built are real hospital first and was ready to start recruiting PHS physicians. As yet that hospital had no internist on staff and there was a debate about whether to allow internists from Dexter to admit patients to their hospital. A lot of local politics.

Some years after my program became the National Heath Service Corps, it was, most unfortunately, largely dismantled. I would bring it back in a minute even though I don't have a sense of its effectiveness. Concerns were raised that most of the physicians stayed in their assigned locations only for the 2 or 3 years of their obligation and then left. The PHS still serves as the umbrella organization for health care for the Indian Health Service and the Bureau of Prisons, but to the best of my knowledge the only remaining medical school scholarship program is in the military. The PHS may have an arrangement whereby doctors agree to work in underserved areas for a specified period and in return part or all of their educational indebtedness is forgiven.

For my obligated service I ended up at the Tri-River Clinic in Uxbridge, Massachusetts. The hope was that I would consider settling there after my 3 years were up since it was a medically underserved rural community. The PHS had opened a practice in a small apartment and had started to construct what became the current clinic. The clinic was going to be operated as part of the University of Massachusetts Medical Center, serving as a site for resident training. Another feature was that it was an hour's drive from Andover— close enough that we could attend family functions but not so close that we couldn't live our own lives.

Three physicians, all employees of the university, worked in the Blackstone Valley, where Uxbridge is located; the area once had five general practitioners, but over time they were lost. The doctors had left for the same reasons that much of rural America has lost its practitioners. Part of it was economics. The area had once been vital, with textile mills and manufacturers of textile machinery, but the industries had migrated to the Carolinas. Also, doctors were no longer training to be general practitioners. When the health center was first created, one part-time person remained.

The community, frustrated in its attempts to recruit doctors, approached the medical school for help. The medical school, which was just starting up, got the region designated as a Health Manpower Shortage Area and qualified as a PHS site. The medical school was interested in appearing to be making good on the promise it had made when it was started: to train primary care doctors. The medical school realized that it would be useful, mainly for the departments of medicine and pediatrics, to have an off-campus, community-based training site where residents could experience primary care. The clinic was going to be staffed with internal medicine and pediatrics practitioners as an alternative to the family practice model. We were going to do it better than family practice because the internists would be better at adult medicine and the pediatricians would be better at children's medicine. The family practice physicians weren't even invited.

The tie to the medical school was part of the reason for my attraction. When you're at the end of your residency, you become apprehensive about cutting the umbilical cord to the university setting, and that can affect where you choose to practice. Because a connection to a university center is conducive to better medicine, it makes it more likely that someone would commit to a career close by. We also had a cooperative arrangement for admitting our patients to the university's hospital, which worked out well. Medical students were less involved than residents. Students came through during their pediatrics rotation for exposure to community-based pediatrics at Tri-River, but in medicine it was an elective.

When I started, I was the only PHS conscriptee. Two internists and two pediatricians were employed by the university, and I was assigned to work with them for my 3-year tour. During my first months I decided that I enjoyed being a primary care internist and was not interested in a cardiology fellowship. In a Health Manpower Shortage Area, you can be a primary care physician and get first crack at everything without a lot of preselection of patients. If a man in Uxbridge has a headache, he doesn't go to a neurologist first; he comes to you, and you decide whether he needs to see a neurologist. It's a different dynamic from that in a more suburban setting.

These days I see about 20 patients a day. I do health maintenance exams in the morning and in the afternoon I see patients for acute illnesses or follow-up. I see a representative adult population with a great range of problems. In some respects it's harder to be a good primary care doctor than a good gastroenterologist or cardiologist. You have to maintain your clinical acumen over a much wider spectrum of diseases. Primary care people are frequently criticized for such things as not having a neurologist see a patient who turns out to have a brain tumor. That can happen and it's terrible, but through experience and learning, and by recognizing the pattern of patients you've seen before, you develop a clinical sense that enables you to make good clinical decisions.

We see many patients with colds, but they have other problems too—some emotional, some medical. They have hypertension, diabetes, chronic bronchitis, arthritis, or ulcers. Having been here for over a decade, I have a large group of people who consider me their doctor. A patient has his or her problems taken care of in one place. I do dermatology too, but not very well. The two areas in which I was most marginally trained were office gynecology and dermatology. Most of what I know, I learned on my own and from short courses.

The best thing about what I do is treat people over a long time and provide continuity of care. The essence of primary care, and of all clinical endeavors, is the long-term relationship with patients. You're their doctor in every sense of the word, and they rely on you for counsel. When my patients are admitted to the university's hospital and their new doctors make recommendations that I don't know about, the patients will talk to me about it before they make a decision—and that's gratifying. I know them not only in a medical sense but in their social and family context. In our community hospital, I take care of a majority of their problems, but when they go to the university setting I'm out of the picture. It is a problem because we are an unused resource. When the new physicians feel strongly about a certain course of action, the patient would feel much more comfortable agreeing to it if the primary care physician were in the loop.

Our exclusion occurs mainly because of carelessness. The person becomes a patient of the university and is seen out of context by physicians who are busy and making decisions of the moment and then going on to something else. No one has the sense of connecting with the person. They don't skip over me for disparaging reasons; after all, I'm on the faculty and teach clinical medicine at the university. They forget. It happens all of the time even within the institution, faculty to faculty.

I am not bothered by being tied to a patient day in and day out, even when the problem is intractable and probably insoluble. Some impossible problems I don't particularly relish. But in a kind of selection process people choose their doctor and their doctor chooses them. I now have a panel of patients that I have worked hard to develop. Like other people in the community, my patients are just plain, solid citizens. They don't come to waste my time. If they have a complaint, there's something wrong with them. If things work out, they're grateful; if things don't turn out as well as they could, they're not vindictive.

Doctors are often most comfortable taking care of people with whom they can identify as peers. I'm a peer to my patients in that we have similar backgrounds. They're like my extended family. As with people who live in the inner cities, we have our share of drug addicts and down-and-outers in the Tri-River service area, and we do the best we can for them. We don't discriminate against them, cast them aside, or refuse to care for them if they can't pay their bills. We do our best, recognizing that we are probably stronger in some settings than in others.

Resolving a patient's problem by a procedure done with one's own two hands, as a surgeon does, unquestionably would be appealing. There is a finality to that as well as a bonding between patient and physician. Patients bond to that person because the trust they have had to place in that practitioner is great, which is different from simply prescribing an antibiotic. Most of our patients are willing to go to our local community facilities for certain problems, but if they need to have surgery, even something as incidental as an appendectomy, they go to a larger facility.

We don't have an emergency room (ER) in our clinic; we send patients with emergencies to a hospital in a nearby small community where they provide a full-time emergency medical staff. Until recent years, most of their ER physicians trained in internal medicine, and the ER director was one of my internal medicine residents. I'm getting gray, and some of the people I trained are now in practice in the community. I teach residents and occasional medical students in our clinic and I do ward rounds for a month or two each year at the medical school. These academic ties have been important to my job satisfaction, but they're not easy to maintain because when I go there for a month my practice doesn't stop.

One of my goals is to let others know that it's a reasonable career objective to become a primary care internist, and I do so by my daily existence. It's funny to think back to when I was a senior resident and the only person in my program not planning a subspecialty fellowship. The reaction from other residents and faculty was that it was terrible to waste such a wonderful mind, but they had been subspecialty-oriented and trained.

I am happy with what I'm doing and I will stay with it, especially if we get a new building for our clinic; we reached the limit of space capacity 3 years ago. Though I manage the clinic, I'm a better doctor than manager. I manage by example. If I need the doctors to see more patients, I'll see more patients and demonstrate that it's possible.

My wife and I have two daughters. The older one is absolutely not interested in medicine. In fact, she spends most of her waking hours feeling phobic about becoming sick. When someone in the family gets sick, she wants to move out of the house until the sick person gets better. As for my younger daughter, I don't know what she will want to do.

I wouldn't discourage a career in medicine. There's an aptitude that you must have, but I can't define it. You must be able to interact with people comfortably and have a scientific orientation. A certain unmeasurable energy is also needed to do it well. Without it, medicine become incredibly burdensome and the doctor becomes disenchanted. I recently went through this with one of my original partners. He was a very good primary care internist but he lost his enthusiasm for what he was doing. It became intolerable, and now he is retraining at the medical school by doing a fellowship in environmental medicine.

To those of us younger people who never knew the halcyon days, medicine is still okay, but there have been changes, even during the time I've been in practice. The interaction with third-party payers, the general audit process of what doctors do, the second guessing and questioning are all facts of life now. I've even participated in the evolution of some of these changes. Initially, when I first became a member of the medical staff at the nearby community hospital, I was received coldly by the other doctors because I was a federal and state employee. They regarded it like a communist incursion into their midst. But in time they began to realize that I wasn't unlike them and I became their president for 2 years. The first year, I was elected unanimously. The second year, I was elected by two votes. The third year, I didn't even run because it was obvious that I would not be reelected. This was because of an action against a long-term practitioner on the staff who did not practice quality medicine and whom we had dismissed from the staff. I was perceived as being responsible for the action and was sued. Even without the law suit it was an unpleasant experience. On the other hand, our action had a positive impact on the quality of care in the hospital.

Past criticism of the profession has a certain validity. A live-and-let-live approach meant that so long as someone didn't tread on your turf, you weren't terribly concerned about whether what he or she did was up to snuff. Partly due to outside influences, but also because the hospital setting has changed greatly, we have a whole new group of people who realize that anything less than optimal reflects on every practitioner in the facility. We're even more sensitive to that at the community hospital than we would be in a university hospital. When an unfortunate outcome occurs at the university, the patient's first thought is, "Well, at least I was at the university." But tolerance of an unfavorable outcome in the community hospital is far lower because the reaction is, "Well, I should have been at the university." The funny thing is that I'm the same practitioner at both places.

Time for family and for self is a universal issue for physicians. The solution for primary care physicians is to practice in groups and have enough partners to allow for time off. In my clinic, we cover for each other and I'm free on my nights off. Yet one of the cardiologists in the neighboring town is on call just about all of the time. Even with my more relaxed time demands, I get complaints from my wife and kids that I'm not home enough. I tell them I'm home more than my colleagues are, but they judge me in terms of other people, such as real (nonphysician) parents.

With respect to more global matters, when it comes to the competing issues of having large geographic regions where huge segments of society have no access to doctors, and of confronting the incredible costs of becoming a physician and the unbelievable indebtedness that students incur, my solution would be to recreate the National Health Service Corps and make every medical school graduate serve in it. Society makes a big investment in the training of a doctor even if the doctor incurs $100,000 of debt because that sum represents just a portion of the total educational costs. Everyone who goes to medical school incurs an obligation to serve for a couple of years in an underserved area. If everyone had to do it, I'm sure that some of the doctors would stay on as assigned. The program would reduce the students' indebtedness and the societal benefits would far outweigh the administrative costs.

Chapter 10

GENERAL PEDIATRICS

Some pediatricians concentrate their efforts on a narrow subset of medical problems, some remain clinical generalists, and some extend their professional activities beyond direct patient care to encompass issues related to the ways in which society as a whole deals with the care and nurturing of children. Dr. DeWitt is in the latter group.

Dr. Thomas G. DeWitt is a general pediatrician. He is professor of pediatrics and family and community medicine in the medical school of the University of Massachusetts Medical Center, Worcester. In addition to seeing patients, he devotes significant time to the training of general pediatricians at the local and national levels.

Thomas G. DeWitt, M.D., General Pediatrics, Academic Medical Center

I learned that I like the way pediatricians think and look at families and communities. A good pediatrician must be aware of the broader impact of society on children because children are disenfranchised and you have to focus on their environment as well as their immediate health problems. . . . What sets the profession apart is the deep intimacy that we have with our patients through our involvement in life and death.

133

I did not become interested in medicine in childhood. There weren't even any physicians in our family. In high school, I wrestled and was active politically. By senior year, I was class president and disengaged from socially conscious political activity. During summers in high school, I worked for a railroad. Mixing with blue collar railroad workers was a profound personal experience in a new culture.

When I went to Amherst College in 1967, I intended to go to business school. College campuses were tumultuous then and there I was, from a conservative background in upstate New York and the midwest. It was a shock to attend a liberal eastern college and encounter a social upheaval. I saw a totally new dimension of people, issues, and concerns. When I went to Amherst, I joined the Young Republicans Club but soon realized that I was on the fringe. I gradually changed my whole way of looking at issues and at people. My social awareness blossomed and I began to think seriously about what I wanted to do in life.

In high school I had done well but had no special area of interest. In an independent study for an advanced science program I had removed a mammary tumor from a mouse. We didn't really know what we were doing. The mouse survived the surgery but died during childbirth 2 days later. I remember it to this day, so maybe that started my interest in pediatrics.

Early in college, I made friends with several premedical students. I saw medicine as intellectually stimulating and with great potential for serving people and addressing challenging issues. Also, it appeared to be a secure profession (it is much less so today), and I didn't want something in which financial security would be a constant problem. During my sophomore year I decided on premed.

I almost flunked the first semester of organic chemistry because I was going through so much turmoil thinking about societal and personal values. I'm not sure just how much organic chemistry has to do with medicine ultimately, but it does test the depth of your commitment. For me, organic chemistry was the turning point that made my decision final.

During one summer vacation I talked to several physicians in my home town about becoming a doctor. In our conversations, I asked why they had gone into medicine. They didn't romanticize and were frank about the time, energy, and sacrifices that go into being a physician. But I got a very real sense that they enjoyed what they were doing. Ironically, one of them was a general surgeon whose daughter I later married. The talks were very helpful.

One of the physicians was an anesthesiologist who had started as a general practitioner. He had presided over a difficult delivery and been deeply upset by the death of the child and the near-death of the mother. It made him take a hard look at staying in medicine. In the end, he switched to anesthesiology. It was interesting to hear him describe his reasoning process.

On subsequent occasions I have turned again to physicians for help with a career decision and I can't remember anyone who was reluctant to talk and to share. They all presented balanced statements and were always eager and encouraging. They helped me to make some difficult decisions and to continue in medicine. One of my major gratifications here is to be of help to students who come to my office in times of depression, say after a particularly hard exam. We talk and more often than not they leave feeling better. I guess I'm trying to pay back for the help I got.

I entered medical school interested in pursuing an area with a lot of patient contact and many possibilities for serving people. I probably had a primary care field in mind but, under strong influence from my surgeon father-in-law, I also loved my surgical rotation. Still, the idea of dealing with public health issues was an underlying influence in my selection of an area of medicine. I never wavered once I made my decision. There must have been some sense of answering to a calling, but I never felt quite that spiritual about it. In the back of my mind issues of politics and of dealing with broad social concerns were tied in.

Various factors attracted me to Rochester Medical School. Many Amherst students had attended there and it had an excellent reputation. Once there I found it to be much more politically conservative than I had realized. I suppose if I had known then what I know now, I might have gone elsewhere.

An influential factor during my first year of medical school was an elective sponsored by the department of pediatrics to provide clinical exposure to balance the traditional curriculum during the first 2 years. The department chairman was active in establishing pediatric outreach and community health programs. The department consisted of an exciting group of faculty who attracted excellent residents. I was assigned to a first-year resident who was an enthusiastic teacher. My time with him was a strong influence in my choosing pediatrics.

I learned that I like the way pediatricians think and look at families and communities. A good pediatrician must be aware of the broader impact of society on children because children are disenfranchised and you have to focus on their environment as well as their immediate health problems. I didn't appreciate it then quite as much as I do now. Rochester's outreach program strongly underscored that concern as well as many other issues that we confront today.

When I picked pediatrics, I was still single. I met my wife between my sophomore and junior years. I think her father was chagrined that I was going into pediatrics. He had the general surgeon's view of pediatricians as nice people who are on the periphery of medicine. Today I try to be a strong spokesperson for pediatrics. Even though our intellectual, clinical, academic, and general abilities are on a par with any other specialty in medicine, pediatrics has been looked down on because of its heavy emphasis on behavior and development, considered by some to be a soft science. Many physicians regard true medicine as biochemical; and when society thinks of medicine, they think of surgeons and internists.

How much you get paid is a reflection of someone's judgment of your worth, and pediatrics has never been high on the reimbursement list. I am encouraged that a shift is occurring and there is a new approach to the specialties. Some have risen in stature and some have slipped, but none is more or less intellectual than before—it's just that outside influences have caused a shift. Orthopedic surgery used to be considered all saws and chisels, but now its techniques are sophisticated and it attracts better students. Internal medicine has declined, not because it is any less intellectual or challenging but because of factors such as AIDS and reimbursement questions. I am biased, but I don't think there has been a shift yet in favor of pediatrics.

However, you should not decide on a field on the basis of its stature within the medical profession. You should pick what you really enjoy and are proud of. That's how I chose pediatrics. At the time, it was respected but not revered. Aside from the intellectual component of my decision, I had a gut feeling that pediatrics was right for me and fitted my way of thinking about medicine.

My view was reinforced in my second year when I worked with a doctor in adolescent medicine who became a mentor during the remainder of medical school. We hit it off early on when I took an elective with her. She was extremely enthusiastic about what she was doing. Afterward, when I did a continuity experience with her in adolescent medicine, she was an avid proponent of my ideas while challenging me in a supportive way.

Nevertheless, as I started my third year, I was not absolutely convinced about pediatrics. After the third-year rotations, it boiled down to surgery or pediatrics. Many people regard them as antithetical but in fact such a choice is not all that uncommon. My final decision was influenced greatly by the personalities I met in the two fields. Most pediatricians are caring, sensitive people who are warm and friendly to their patients. I certainly saw surgeons, such as my father-in-law, who displayed those attributes, but there were too many who didn't have them or didn't display them, and that was a major factor for me.

In the end, I felt that I wanted to be in an environment where I would like most of my immediate colleagues. I thought that I would rather be outside of surgery and pick the surgeons that I liked rather than being in surgery and having constantly to vary my dealings with people based on personality types. Also, I was tired of studying and I liked the thought of 3 years of training in pediatrics as opposed to 5 in surgery. Ironically, once in pediatrics I ended up doing 6 years of postgraduate training—3 as a resident, 1 as chief resident, and 2 as a fellow.

As much for personal as for academic reasons (I was getting married between my third and fourth years and wanted to spend time with my wife-to-be, who was still in college in Washington, D.C.), I accepted a 1-year fellowship after my second year of medical school. In working with my mentor, I had become interested in health services, personnel, and support systems for chronically ill and dying adolescents. With people at Rochester, I designed a 1-year study related to that issue at Children's Hospital in Washington, D.C.

Once in Washington, I ran into a brick wall. I was permitted to follow the patients as a clinical elective but not to study them even though my project only involved filling out questionnaires. I couldn't figure out the problem—maybe it was that I was an outsider and a medical student without a local advisor. Some of it was due to the hospital staff's possessiveness regarding the patients and a general feeling that one ought not to talk to dying kids about dying. Now there's a lot more openness and I'm sure I could have done the study today. Back then, I ended up doing largely the same work but with adolescent diabetics in an adolescent clinic. Their doctors were much more receptive to my talking to their patients.

Dying adolescent patients terrified even the pediatricians, whereas the diabetics did not. So I spent my year looking at psychological parameters in diabetic control. It was my first break in a continuum of education and it gave me time to reinforce my choice of pediatrics. It also laid the groundwork for my later interest in academic medicine. Some students go to work for a year after college and enter medical school with a better perspective, and I endorse that. It's difficult to arrange for something like that during your residency years, and by then you've made a reasonably firm commitment to a field.

I used my last year in medical school to round out my education. I designed a well-balanced program but it did include a subinternship in pediatrics. I didn't give much thought to any pediatric subspecialty since that decision usually comes during residency. You pick your residency with a view toward its ability to help you get into a good fellowship program afterward but not on the basis of whether you plan to become a gastroenterologist or a primary care physician. I went to Yale because I thought it was one of the best residency programs I interviewed. It provided balanced general pediatric training, whereas the program at Children's Hospital in Boston seemed too fragmented. I wanted a program with close comradeship, interpersonal goodwill, and real caring about residents as individuals and about their education. I also felt that I probably wanted to go into academic medicine. In addition, my wife was accepted to Yale's divinity school. Initially we intended after completing our training programs to go back to te midwest where Yale's reputation would help each of us to find a good job. Although it is helpful to train where you're planning to settle, it's also important to train in a program with a national reputation that will open doors and allow you to get into a good fellowship in the place where you want to settle.

Like any residency, the 3 years at Yale were a stressful challenge. In some ways I'm pleased with the new regulations restricting working hours for residents. During my first 3 months, we were on call 5 nights a week and in the hospital 140 hours out of the 168. I appreciated the good comradeship—we really supported each other. The greatest emotional stress occurred after the internship. The second year was easier and it allowed me to see what hell I had gone through. One of the more difficult times in my marriage was after the first year when we looked at each other across the table as strangers because my wife was in divinity school and I was immersed in the hospital. We experienced a decompression or posttraumatic syndrome, something not uncommon after intense rotations.

Today residents don't spend as much time on call, but I'm concerned about the intensity of the illnesses they see. Patients spend less time in the hospital, but instead of one terminal patient a resident will have four or five incredibly ill kids. In pediatrics easy problems don't come to the hospital, only the complex, very serious problems. That's true also in internal medicine where patients have HIV and cancer.

Your experiences in pediatrics have a tremendous impact on you. From my internship year I can still remember my first patient to die. I gave him morphine as he was writhing in pain and I had to wonder whether the morphine may have hastened things. Yet from those experiences—and I remember every death—has emerged a deeper understanding of what medicine is all about, about life and death and even religion, and about medicine as a calling.

Seeing life and death as a doctor is an intimate entree into people's lives. As a pediatrician, I'm there at births and, sadly, at the end of some young people's lives. The meaningfulness of that is hard to convey. I have helped families work through their grieving even before their children have died. Those relationships are at the core of medicine. There's the intellectualism, knowing the science that goes into treating illness, and there are the surgical-technical skills (pediatricians must acquire some of them, what with IVs and spinal taps), but what sets the profession apart is the deep intimacy that we have with our patients through our involvement in life and death. That was not as clear to me as a medical student as it was when I was a resident.

In contrast to some observers, I don't see a major decline in the caring aspects of medicine. I am encouraged by the physicians and the medical students I work with here. I almost sense a resurgence of caring, although there is a real danger of being drawn into the finances and politics of medicine. That medicine is going through difficult financial times may turn out to be a boon by discouraging the entry of people who want to make a lot of money and by attracting more of the idealistic and altruistic people. I feel bad about these difficult times and I'm getting caught up in them, but they may result in medicine becoming more humane and reinforce what people feel was lost during the past couple of decades.

But I'm digressing. When I became the chief resident in pediatrics, my wife had one more year of hard work at the divinity school, but it was one of the best years of my life. A chief resident plays a significant role in the wonderful world between the faculty and the residents, and he or she tries to make things work well. I loved it. It was a year for a lot of personal and clinical growth. Since I saw almost all of the pediatrics patients, I was exposed to a tremendous variety of clinical problems. I got to know many members of the faculty in a way that I never quite knew them as a resident. My wife was pregnant toward the end of that year and during the beginning of my fellowship year. All in all, it was a very happy time.

During my senior year of residency, I became interested in gastroenterology and have since then done research on diarrhea and oral rehydration. I interviewed with programs in gastroenterology and was on the verge of applying for fellowship training when I received a Robert Wood Johnson General Academic Fellowship. I spent the first year of the fellowship at Yale, mainly in classes on epidemiology methodology and statistics. I did a project in clinical decision making and acute diarrhea. I was trying to become a clinical researcher. I had done just enough during my clinical research year in medical school to know what I didn't know, and this program gave me skills I was lacking.

During the first year of fellowship I did 3 hours of course work a day and 18 hours of homework, and I loved it. I took statistics, computer work, methodology, case-control studies, controlled trials, and cross-sectional surveys. I also started the clinical project I mentioned. The second year had some course work, but there was more clinical research and you were expected to emerge as a well-trained academic general pediatrician.

Then I came here to head general pediatrics and the pediatric outpatient service. When I came here I hadn't the foggiest idea of what I had become professionally. Over the years, however, people have tapped into the training I received during the fellowship and I have become a resource for those who want to look at clinical questions. After 9 years, I'm here to stay in general pediatrics. The environment and my chairman are very good, and national and local developments allow me to pursue general academic pediatrics and primary care issues here as well as anywhere else.

How I spend my time depends on the crisis for the week. I do a fair amount of general pediatrics by following some 500 patients in several weekly clinic sessions. Based in a tertiary care center, we probably have a higher percentage of chronically ill, complex children than do practitioners on the outside. Unlike some academic generalists, I don't focus on any specific disease entity. My interest is very much in looking at clinical and practice issues for the pediatrician generalist and the chronic care pediatrician. When I interact with pediatricians on the outside, I understand what they're talking about.

I see my patients just the way a pediatrician does on the outside. In our group we cover for each other when someone's away. I round on the ward 1 month a year and in the newborn nursery 1 month a year. I also take general pediatric night call about once a week and do nursery rounds on the weekends. I teach medical students in different courses and settings, and I cover medical interviewing, epidemiology, and physical diagnosis. I also see students as an advisor.

I'm not doing as much clinical research as I would like, but I am writing a proposal for a major research grant for looking at primary care and clinical outcomes. When I came here, I was assigned many administrative, clinical, and training responsibilities that diverted my attention from research. As I've moved along, I've divested myself of some duties and hope to return to research.

I don't have as much time for my own children as I would like. They are 10, 7, and 4. When I was a resident, someone said, "Of the three F's—fame, fortune, and free time for family—you can have only two." I'm not sure you can even have two. My life is pretty much divided between my clinical career, my academic work, and my family. I do very little else on my own. Any sports or other activities revolve around my family. Any socializing revolves around my professional life or my children as they relate to other families. One of the main struggles in academic medical life is to achieve balance, and I've given up research, at least up to now. As for personal growth, my family and my medical experiences have made me a more tolerant person. I did some pottery when I was a resident but not since then; sailing is another neglected love.

It's too early to tell whether any of my children will go into medicine, but I would be delighted if they did. I talk to them about medicine, but I probably should do more. Sometimes they come on rounds with me, depending on their mood and which of their friends are available. As I tell my students, the important thing for me has been to make my career decisions based on what would fit with my own philosophical approach to life and people, and to avoid compromising idealism. If you really like what you're doing, and feel that you aren't ignoring who you are and what you feel comfortable doing, then you can make most of your decisions work in a medical career. The catch is that I'm still exploring those dimensions of myself. I encourage students to seek out people and ask hard questions. There's wisdom out there that one can tap into, but sometimes you have to force people to sit down, slow up, and talk.

Students should not be too frenetic about the choice of a clinical discipline. Depending on how thoroughly you have come to terms with yourself, you can do well in any number of different fields. There is a whole spectrum of opportunities within each area. For example, although you may think you are closing doors when you choose pediatrics, it presents many possibilities. I could practice pediatrics. I could become a hospital administrator. I could even go into clinical research. You should not feel that once you've made a choice, you can never take a different tack. Remember the physician back home to whom I turned for advice, the one who had switched into anesthesiology from clinical practice? When he changed direction, he had a family and was well along in his career. It was helpful to talk to him and see that even in midcareer he still had the option to make a major change. Who knows, I could yet become a surgeon!

Chapter 11

GENERAL SURGERY

Although some surgeons would prefer to remain generalists, the tides of academe and the demands of the clinical discipline pressure many of them into a specialty. Dr. Wertheimer tried to resist, but he moved almost inexorably from general surgery into a field of concentration.

Dr. Michael D. Wertheimer is a surgeon who devotes a major fraction of his time to the surgical treatment of breast cancer and to clinical research on the treatment of the disease. He is a professor of surgery in the school of medicine of the University of Massachusetts Medical Center in Worcester and he is the director of the Breast Center.

Michael D. Wertheimer, M.D., Surgery,
Academic Medical Center

At one time in health care, we valued the doctor–patient relationship as paramount. As doctors became more specialized, they gained more and more intellectual satisfaction from the disease rather than from health or, in some situations, even from the patient. That shifted the focus away from the humanism of the profession. . . . My take-home message is that there's still a great deal of joy to be derived from the practice of medicine. Like most of the physicians I know, when I get past some of the irritations of practicing in today's heavily regulated health care system, I love what I do.

I drifted into medicine without making a definite decision about it. The seed didn't come from any family role model. I am a first-generation American and no one in my immediate family ever finished high school. I was impressed with my pediatrician who made house calls. I majored in science and was interested but had no great affinity for it. Corny as it sounds, I was attracted to medicine by the humanism—the interpersonal relationships. Working in a specialty and having an academic career were afterthoughts. In college I never considered any serious alternatives to medicine, although my father wanted me to go into a small family business.

When I got to medical school, surgery had a romance and intrigue about it. Almost immediately, I met several role models who were doing adult and pediatric cardiac surgery, and I spent time in their animal lab working on heart transplantation. I was also exposed to operations on infants with congenital heart disease. It was so overpowering that I said, "This is it."

I did consider other areas, but I must have felt an affinity for the surgical lifestyle and for the dynamism of the things surgeons did. At the same time, and this has caused conflict for me, I felt that I was really different from most surgeons. For example, I did well enough in psychiatry and obstetrics to consider those fields even though others pointed out how unusual it was to be choosing between psychiatry and surgery. I reached my decision without a lot of deliberation.

Surgery is a little like being in the marines, with a very top-down hierarchy and with rigid and prescribed behavior and demands of the training. If you can't accept that and fit in, it can be painful. That was an issue for me for a long time and, to some extent, it still is because my values with respect to my personal life and the way I feel about patients and family are somewhat different from those of the average surgeon, if there is such a thing.

I was the first chief resident here when this was a new medical school. I have been on the faculty ever since. My professional work has evolved over the years and gradually I've become somewhat subspecialized into an interest in cancer of the breast, although I still do other kinds of surgery. For many different reasons, narrowing of focus is perhaps inevitable in a university practice, but I always preferred being a generalist. I continue to perform trauma surgery and some general surgery and love those aspects of being a surgical generalist.

In breast cancer, where I spend most of my time now, the residents jokingly refer to me as a "psychiatrist with a knife." Patients with breast cancer, as do most other sick people, require compassion, understanding, time, process, conversation, and empathy. But many surgeons love the operating room (OR) and would be happy to be there day and night—in some instances to the exclusion of everything else. They would be pleased if others screened the patients and delivered them to the OR and they just did "cases."

At one time in health care, we valued the doctor–patient relationship as paramount. As doctors became more specialized, they gained more and more intellectual satisfaction from the disease rather than from health or, in some situations, even from the patient. That shifted the focus away from the humanism of the profession. Even some internists look on a patient's problem as a "disease," much the way some surgeons look on a patient as a "procedure." This pernicious tendency abstracts medicine and depersonalizes the patient. Yet I believe that more doctors are becoming sensitive to the humanism again, and I feel that pendulum swinging back.

Every patient with an illness, especially a surgical one, is frightened and anxious and needs compassion, time, and someone with whom to talk. In a surgical situation, that is the responsibility of the surgeon more than anyone else. It doesn't matter initially whether it's to be a short-term or long-term intervention; there is a right way to care for sick human beings and it should be uniform.

I love doing surgery and treating surgical diseases. Even after 20 years, it's exhilarating and a source of pride. Surgeons rarely retire willingly from active practice or hate to get up in the morning to go to the hospital. Even simple surgical problems give an immediate gratification that's hard to achieve in other fields of medicine. Most of us truly love the work. The drama of cardiac surgery first drew me into surgery, but later, when I lived as a resident in cardiac surgery, I realized that it was not the lifestyle I wanted. At the same time, I started experiencing the delights of simpler surgical practice.

To go into cardiac surgery, I needed 5 years of training in general surgery first, so I applied for that. But I also applied for a residency in ob/gyn and couldn't decide which one I wanted. I had become interested in ob/gyn because the chairman at Penn was probably the most charismatic individual on the faculty. He is a wonderful person and a powerful role model, and I have kept in touch with him. I was excited to be accepted into his program. Ob/gyn had a lot of interesting surgery in it and I might have been happy in that field; who knows? But when I was accepted in general surgery at the Beth Israel Hospital in Boston, I turned down ob/gyn.

Later, after my second year of residency, when I was feeling shell-shocked by the rigors of the day-to-day demands of surgical residency, I reapplied to Penn's ob/gyn program, prepared to leave surgery. What got to me were the time demands, the hierarchical culture, and many other things — all at an intensity I had never experienced. Once again, I was accepted to Penn's ob/gyn program. I held on to that acceptance for a time and almost bailed out of surgery. Finally, I decided to stick with surgery and the head of ob/gyn wished me luck.

In medical school I had spent a lot of time on various surgical services. Between my third and fourth years, I went to England to work under a renowned cardiac surgery team, but it was very different from what I was to encounter later in the residency. Maybe it was the social isolation. I had recently married and my wife and I were in a new city, Boston, without family or many friends. The was little or no sympathy or understanding of the personal trials and tribulations that surgical residents experience. The stresses were different, and probably quantitatively greater by virtue of the time commitment, from those of residents in internal medicine, pediatrics, or psychiatry, and the situation hasn't changed much today. In the early 1970s, there were weeks when I never left the hospital. That had a bad effect on personal and family life and personality development.

I toughed out the residency for a while and then, after 3 years, decided to leave the program to take time off, do different things, and rethink my plans. Around that time, I met Dr. Wheeler, who had come here to start the surgery department at the new medical school. He hired me as the first chief resident and gave me an immediate year's leave of absence.

For 6 months I worked for Caesar Chavez in a clinic for migrant farm workers in California. I had been active in such things in the past. Surgery, perhaps even more than internal medicine or some other fields, is very much a cross-cultural skill. With surgical training you can practice anywhere, whether you know the language or the culture or not, and do good by relieving suffering. That was what I wanted to experience and I did. It was like practicing third-world medicine.

Mostly I helped a volunteer physician run a general medicine clinic. I was midway in my training so I wasn't prepared to practice surgery, but we did deliver babies in the clinic. I performed some surgery in the clinic and in the local hospital on patients who were excluded from the health care system and were not welcome at the hospital except for emergencies. My wife, who was then a medical student, worked there too. The experience affected me in the way that any deep, personal relationship with people who badly need your help can change your life. That's the appeal that medicine has always had for me and the part that has been lacking in my university career.

I was the first chief resident in surgery in this medical school during its pioneer days. We were setting up new programs and it was a great adventure. As the institution matured, my practice did too. I ended up getting pigeonholed in a defined clinical area, partly because we developed so many subspecialists who now do so many of the things that I once did, and partly because you are expected to become an expert and to do research and write. That usually involves going deeper and focusing more narrowly in a few areas. For me it ended up being breast cancer as a special clinical interest, although I do other things.

During my residency training, I did not continue in cardiac surgery because the work became incompatible with my vision of later life in a surgical career. Besides, almost everyone I knew professionally in that field was angry, arrogant, and abusive. I didn't need the high drama any more; general surgery was more satisfying. I never even applied for cardiac surgery because, with a few exceptions such as urology, orthopedics, and ophthalmology, to enter the mainstream programs of general surgery—thoracic, vascular, cardiac—you don't apply until your fourth or fifth year of general training, and before I reached that point I had decided to move ahead in general surgery and see where it led.

Today general surgery is virtually extinct. When I went into it, it was still a well-defined area. There were many centers where you could be a true general surgeon. You did major abdominal surgery, some thoracic and vascular surgery, and limited gynecology, orthopedics, and urology, depending on the environment.

At around the beginning of my fifth residency year, I decided that I didn't want to prolong my training any longer. I wanted to continue learning on my own. In retrospect, it probably would have been good to get more training. But during my final year the chairman offered me a faculty position as a general surgeon. The department needed generalists because they're the backbone of a teaching program.

I never considered private practice. Academic medical life seemed to come as close to a pure form of practice as one could hope to find in that there were fewer financial constraints on the kinds of patients you can see. I was happy never knowing who did or did not pay my bill and being free to see any mix of patients, including poor people with no insurance. This has changed, though. Now we receive financial profiles on patients and the hospital tries to influence us to improve the bottom line. Despite these trends, my practice remains blind to this, which is hard to do in private practice.

Starting out today, I could not evolve into a general surgeon. Nearly everyone does subspecialty training and gains a high level of skill in a narrowly focused type of surgery or in relation to a specific organ. Subspecialists have expertise in areas that general surgeons used to cover, and here we have someone in each area who knows a lot more than I do. I still have a role, but a general surgeon couldn't come in now and function as I do. In the last 10 years, we have hired only subspecialists, which is good and bad. No question, subspecialists are technically skillful and often have better records with lower morbidity and mortality in specific operations. But the disadvantage regarding the decreasing continuity of clinical care in a fragmented system of subspecialists causes patients to suffer in many profound ways.

I try to see my patients holistically, trite as it sounds. You can't be someone's doctor if you regard them as an organ or a procedure. I expose students to this attitude by having them meet patients in clinic who are scheduled to be admitted later for surgery, then to see the patients in the hospital, and then to make house calls afterward whenever possible. This approach to training is getting lost. The role models are the subspecialists, which isn't the best frame of reference.

My practice is dominated by referrals of patients with breast cancer. It still includes trauma and general abdominal surgery, but I'm identified with surgical oncology. I'm accredited by the Society of Surgical Oncology because of my experience. To do surgical oncology today, you must commit much of your time to basic research. Since I was drawn to medicine mainly by its clinical and interpersonal aspects rather than its science, I would not be happy in a major research endeavor. From a purely academic standpoint, even clinical research is probably considered second best. I haven't published as much as I would have liked, and in a university there's little prestige or advancement to be derived from doing mainly clinical care. I did limit my academic activity and productivity somewhat while my children were young so that I could be an involved parent.

I have recently been promoted to professor of surgery and have taken on additional administrative responsibilities in the hospital. That is a common scenario for university physicians as their careers mature. The change and added diversity is very stimulating and one of the wonderful aspects of academic life.

The issues confronting today's students are complex, but they boil down to knowing yourself, knowing which people, activities, and tempo fit best with your personality, and knowing what is intellectually interesting to you. When medicine was wide open and the disciplines and geographic areas were not oversupplied, you determined your heart's desire and sought it out. These days most specialties are overfilled and most cities are exploding with specialists, so you can no longer do anything you want anywhere you want. Sure, you need to take into account personal and psychological issues, but you should try to anticipate and prepare for what the practice of medicine will be like in 10 or 20 years in a rapidly changing health care environment.

Even with a clear idea of the field you want and with a great mentor, your well-considered decision could turn sour because of other constraints. For example, you may decide that you want to be an ophthalmologist in the Boston area where your family resides but learn that it is impossible to make a living in that overcrowded field in a city like Boston. But if you stay flexible regarding geography, you stand a better chance of picking your field. The current emphasis on primary care will also tend to greatly influence training and career options in the future.

For good advice about current constraints, students must first realize that the question needs to be asked. Useful information can be gained by talking to a lot of people and seeking out mentors. If at all possible, start during the first year of medical school, even if the clinical faculty appears formidable. By the time you reach the third-year clerkships, when you are thrown together with faculty on more collegial terms, it may be a little late.

First- and second-year students should take the initiative to gain clinical experience. The best way for a student to begin to understand medicine is to try on his or her own—and I recognize that it's extremely difficult—to experience what illness means from the patient's and the physician's standpoint and to appreciate the impact of a disease on the individual and the family. I would ask a preceptor to assign a patient to a student for several years and require the student to go to the home, come to the doctor's office, or visit the hospital and share whatever that patient is experiencing over time. Then I would have the student write a short story about the experience.

Until you encounter human suffering and learn what a doctor can do to relieve it through the wonderful dynamics of interpersonal relations and technical skills, you will miss the essence of what it means to be a physician or a surgeon. Until then, it's all abstract. An added abstraction comes from seeing specialty medicine in the university setting, which is mainly what third-year students experience. This rarefied exposure doesn't much help students make correct choices for the right reasons. Most students trained at university hospitals see primarily hospitalized patients, which reveals only a small snapshot in time, maybe only 10 percent of what's important about an illness. Absent the human experiences and the continuity, the student is swept up by overly intellectual, academic, political, and other aspects of patient care that abound in a university hospital. Much of this has nothing to do with patients, but what you eventually do as a doctor can be greatly influenced by how you see it.

If your instinct and motivations for going into medicine are in the true Hippocratic and humanitarian traditions, it matters little what specialty you pick. If your feelings for human suffering and your desire to relieve that suffering are your main motivations in medicine, your specialty becomes much less important because you can achieve those goals in any field.

My take-home message is that there's still a great deal of joy to be derived from the practice of medicine. Like most of the physicians I know, when I get past some of the irritations of practicing in today's heavily regulated health care system, I love what I do. Clinical medicine is still a wonderful calling.

Over the last 10 or 15 years, I've been maturing in my practice. In surgery, at least, it takes 5 or 10 years to hit your stride and develop a sense of clinical wisdom. I've learned a great deal about myself and about doctoring from having been deeply involved in raising my two children over the last number of years than from any other experience. It made me more open to other people's needs and to the suffering of patients. The way we treat other people—children, spouses, secretaries, nurses, colleagues—is one and the same, requiring the same skills and sensitivities as does the treatment of our patients. To be a successful physician you must become a satisfied and happy person. You cannot look on it as an academic exercise. That's the conflict that a lot of us experience, certainly around universities.

A career in clinical surgery doesn't necessarily preclude having a family and other interests, but making time for my children took a lot of determination. When our first child was born, my wife was an intern and I had just started out in practice. My schedule wasn't all that full and to some extent I was "Mr. Mom" for the first couple of years. My behavior was considered eccentric and outside the surgeon stereotype, but I'm glad I did it then and continue to be there now for the children. When both parents are in medicine, they need all kinds of outside support—day care, housekeepers, and so forth. Parenting adds enormously to the stress and the pressure of a medical career.

I would neither encourage nor discourage my children from going into medicine. They would have to feel it as a calling. Medicine will never return to what it was, and that may be good because some of the old economic incentives were perverse and may be gone forever. The backlash may be positive in that now only the truly committed and idealistic will want to become physicians. If it works out that way, and I see slight hints of this in the attitudes of our first-year students, that will be very positive.

Chapter 12

INFECTIOUS DISEASES

In the first segment of her career, Dr. Cheeseman worked as a specialist who was called in by other physicians to help them manage a patient with a severe or complicated infection. With the advent of the HIV era, she has continued in that role but she has also become more and more a general practitioner for a circumscribed group of patients, the victims of HIV infection.

Dr. Sarah H. Cheeseman is professor of medicine, microbiology, and pediatrics in the medical school of the University of Massachusetts Medical Center at Worcester. She is an advocate for AIDS clinical trials and sees HIV patients at the medical school's clinics and hospital.

**Sarah H. Cheeseman, M.D., Infectious Diseases,
Academic Medical Center**

By shifting into HIV work as my predominant activity, I now care for patients who do not look forward to an optimistic outcome whereas before I could intervene and save a life or make someone feel a lot better. I think about that a lot. Actually, when you treat someone who knows they have an ultimately fatal disease, and when you give them back quality of life, even if neither of you knows for how long, they are extremely grateful, and you feel a very strong sense of accomplishment.

You won't believe it, but I was in the fifth grade when I decided to become a specialist in infectious diseases. My father wanted me to become a diplomat, but my mother said I was not diplomatic enough. I also thought about becoming an architect. Once in fifth grade when I was assigned to lead a committee planning project, I told my group that we would design a colonial house and not just some popsicle stick model. I told them that if I was going to do all of the work, we would do it my way. The teacher quickly pulled me off the committee and sat me in front of a book in the library with a solitary assignment to read it and give a report to the class. The book was *Microbe Hunters*, by Paul de Kruif, and I reported on Semmelweiss and puerperal fever.

That was it. From then on, there was no question in my mind that I would be a physician in the field of infectious diseases. I read a lot more of medical history. We lived near Johns Hopkins and my dad and I bought memoirs of nearly every doctor from Johns Hopkins. Later I had some wonderful medical school teachers in infectious diseases both in Boston and in Wisconsin.

Because the University of Wisconsin rejected me, I started medical school at Harvard, even though my fiancé was in Wisconsin working on his PhD. During my first year at Harvard, I spent a lot of time with the dean of students trying to effect my transfer to Wisconsin. I even thought of switching to a PhD program in microbiology at Wisconsin. I didn't want to ask my fiancé to move to Boston because Harvard did not have a good reputation in his field of mathematics and I never thought to ask him to take second best. Finally, I got into Wisconsin and transferred there for the last 3 years of medical school. Then I returned to Boston for residency training.

The digression to Wisconsin had pluses and minuses. Harvard was a wonderful place. The students were close as a class and the lectures were stimulating. In Wisconsin, because of curriculum differences, I had to repeat several subjects and also missed a few. For example, I have never taken medical school virology or parasitology. I'm now a clinical virologist and have to cram hard for the parasitology parts of the boards I take.

The Wisconsin students seemed more dependent on their books, and sometimes the lecturers presented outdated concepts. We had been spoon-fed at Harvard and it had been high-quality spoon feeding, but for future life, since we all have to become self-educating, perhaps Wisconsin was better. The people in my Harvard class felt that my going to Wisconsin improved my chances of getting an internship in Boston, and indeed, I was admitted to the Mass. General for house staff training.

The return to Boston posed a dilemma for my husband. As a result of our opting to go there, he did not finish his PhD and changed his field. Part of the reason for the switch was that he found that life was not all that nice out there in academic mathematics. But I have to take some responsibility for the fact that moving away from his thesis advisor was a major blow to his continuing his work. So each of us faced a difficult career decision along the way.

The big choice I had to make was whether to train in internal medicine or pediatrics because either one would have been an entree into infectious disease. I enjoyed them both in medical school— perhaps pediatrics a little more than medicine. During my third-year pediatrics clerkship, an internal medical resident who was rotating through pediatrics and who was my intern was severely reprimanded for treating a patient in status epilepticus with intravenous diazepam. In internal medicine it was regarded as a new but proper thing to do, but its acceptance had not yet filtered into pediatrics. The child did well but the associated furor introduced me to the delay in accepting new therapies in pediatrics, due mainly to concerns about potential effects on growth and development and about unusual metabolism of drugs, a problem seen primarily in very young children. It also reflects an innate clinical conservatism. It was made clear that just because a drug worked in adults, a doctor could not go ahead and adopt it in pediatrics.

The episode was an overwhelming focus of discussion on the pediatric service for several weeks and the medical resident was surprised that something like that could cause such an uproar. She was a good friend and her experience had a lasting effect on me. I concluded that if I went into pediatrics I would always be some years behind in my ability to apply new advances, and so I chose to train in medicine even though I knew that in the future I would want to practice my specialty with children as well as adults.

I still do a great deal with pediatric infectious disease, including several months a year of pediatric infectious disease consults. The choice of a field of residency training doesn't necessarily lock you in for life to one circumscribed area of medicine, but you have to do things to keep pathways open. Even though I had decided to apply for a residency in medicine, I spent most of my fourth year doing pediatric electives because I wasn't going to get much exposure to it in my residency.

Today students seem to take many of their electives in the field in which they want to train so they can demonstrate their abilities and prepare for their residency training. Back then, it did not seem risky for me to work in pediatrics when I was planning to apply for a medical residency. Nobody at Wisconsin gave much thought to getting into a prestigious internship. When students ask for my advice, I suggest they do what I did because in many ways the fourth year of medical school is your last chance. However, few students follow my advice.

I did not spend any time at the hospital where I wanted my residency because from Wisconsin it was difficult to arrange to visit hospitals on the East Coast for a month. I had to rely on having done reasonably well in medical school and on being "different"—a westerner. All this means is it's okay to be yourself. You may not necessarily be handicapped by making choices that are for your education as opposed to choices designed to impress boards and committees.

Even so, I advise my fourth-year students who want to try for a residency at a competitive hospital to spend a month there to evaluate how they will rank in comparison to the current house staff and to create a good impression without relying entirely on recommendation letters and transcripts. But a student has to design the fourth-year schedule during the third year, which necessitates picking the field for training by spring of the third year.

The choice of academic medicine over private practice was a late one for me. It came when I finished my second year of training. I knew that eventually I had to take an infectious disease fellowship but felt vague about what I would do after that. I chose to do a fellowship that included research because during medical school I had the opportunity to serve on a Food and Drug Administration advisory committee and observe how people in infectious disease brought their laboratory experience to clinical issues such as drug licensing. I saw how good people applied what they learned from being laboratory scientists and clinicians, and I decided to get some experience in laboratory research even though I didn't expect to enjoy or make a career of it.

When I finished my fellowship, I had to stay in the Boston area because my husband had accepted a job, and the business world doesn't look favorably on making changes every 2 years. When I came to Worcester, I told my chief that I did not know whether I would make a go of bench research as an independent investigator and didn't even know whether I cared, but I would make a genuine effort. Years later, when we reviewed my record, we decided that I had voted with my feet. I moved off the tenure track and recast my laboratory research into a more clinical mold.

At the time, we were beginning to see HIV infection in Worcester, and my growing outpatient responsibilities rapidly became oriented to HIV. This led to another kind of investigational career, one for which my fellowship research had trained me. I could return to what I was best prepared for: running clinical trials. My fellowship research project had involved a clinical trial, and I gradually settled into academic life as a clinician.

Until HIV, infectious disease practice in a teaching hospital required seeing primarily acute illness with little opportunity for long-term ties to the patients. There were some chronic infections like chronic osteomyelitis, but often those people "belonged" to an orthopedic surgeon. HIV has changed the face of infectious disease. Before that came along, I thought I was happy. I liked the knotty problems and enjoyed seeing only difficult patients—only those who required the full brunt of my subspecialty training. I got my positive reinforcement from the collegial feelings that I had with the physicians I consulted for, particularly the surgeons.

As for balancing my life, until a year ago I thought I was doing well. I tried not to do anything late at night that would keep me from going home unless it had to do with patient care. The diseases for which we can do the most are hyperacute conditions such as meningitis. It's foremost among diseases that strike at any hour of the day or night and require an immediate response. So just because I have a consulting specialty, my hours are no less unpredictable than those of other doctors. These days when I have the equivalent of a large private practice with HIV-infected persons, I take night and weekend speaking engagements because the more you learn about this disease the more committed you become to its prevention and to educating the public. I also feel that with my children approaching their teens, perhaps my commitment to this work says more to them than direct lectures.

But when I added a substantial amount of administrative work, the balance tipped too far. To do everything, I have given up a significant portion of time that I was saving for my family. It's also harder because two of our kids have entered high school and spend less time at home. Now I have to take pains to grab the precious hour with them, and I'm not sure how well it's working or whether it harms the children. At least two thirds of the time I don't get home in time for dinner.

We have a nanny who cooks, cleans, does laundry, and chauffeurs kids. I absolutely could not do it any other way. I don't know whether it would have been different in another specialty. I think some of it is governed by personality. I know people who work with infectious disease in a more time-controlled manner than I do.

By shifting into HIV work as my predominant activity, I now care for patients who do not look forward to an optimistic outcome whereas before I could intervene and save a life or make someone feel better. When you treat someone who knows that he or she has a fatal disease, and when you give that person back quality of life, even if neither of you knows for how long, the person is extremely grateful, and you feel a strong sense of accomplishment. Patients with HIV infection generally know what they're up against, and so patients and physicians appreciate whatever gains are made.

This is different from what you run up against as an infectious disease consultant. Frequently you will treat someone with a devastating infection who hasn't the slightest notion that the infection could have been fatal or permanently disabling. Most patients aren't afraid of infection, and physicians aren't very candid about the threat that an infection poses. For example, when patients are diagnosed with endocarditis, most of them don't realize that it was 100 percent fatal in the preantibiotic era and today has a better than 10 percent mortality rate, even under the best of circumstances. I'm not even confident that doctors themselves appreciate the severity of the infectious diseases we treat.

But it's different with the HIV patients through the whole gamut of challenges—from curing their pneumocystis and getting them back to work, to recognizing that the time has come for chronic pain medication and having a family tell you, "We haven't seen his real personality for months, but now that he's on morphine we can enjoy being with him as a nice person. What a gift for these last few weeks." It's similar with a patient who has been homeless for years and enters a hospice.

I have learned that the more humanistic aspects of medicine, such as giving prolonged care and being satisfied with less than miraculous interventions, are gratifying. Another point is that sharing a meaningful, albeit brief, part of a person's life is an experience that not too many people have. Patients with cancer have a lot of support available; people with AIDS don't. They don't have many people with whom they can be open. I like the fact that our patients will just walk into our clinic and sit down and talk when something's happened to them; they know it's a place where someone will listen. I make the time to talk, but we also have a team of nurse practitioners and a social worker with whom I work closely and we all get to know what sort of things each of us would say. I take secondary gratification from the patient interactions that I can have via the team. After all, doctors don't hang the antibiotics on the IV poles either.

I suspect people are willing to stay in fields where they care for patients with such chronic diseases as arthritis, pulmonary disease, cancer, and geriatric problems because they derive similar gratifications. In HIV, though, we cover everything—life-threatening complications that we can treat successfully and conditions for which we can offer only palliative measures. To be a happy physician, you need to realize that even surgeons, who derive much of their gratification from having the chance to cure, often don't totally cure. In clinical medicine if you can't find pleasure in management and alleviation, then you spend your professional life feeling unfulfilled and frustrated.

My field is a labor-intensive, low-tech, purely cognitive specialty. We have no procedures for which we can bill and other disciplines regard us mainly as pests. We often ask people to do a lot of extra work—draw cultures, look at X-rays, review the Gram stain and the CAT scan, and so on. For other specialties, such as surgery, we usually represent a clinical problem because their needing us means they've run into a serious complication. It takes a lot of work to manage these relationships so the others see us as helpful and not adversarial.

A question I'm asked frequently in relation to choosing infectious disease as a specialty is whether I'm concerned about contracting a disease or taking it home, and whether the dangers of being in my field are different from those of any other specialty. I think the dangers are less than in surgery. Indeed, the only times I worried about it were when I was pregnant. When I realized that I wanted to do virology, I thought I should put it off until I had finished having kids. Then I decided that you can't go back and do another postdoc 5 years later; it's now or never, so you have to be as careful as possible. And during my fellowship, when I was scheduling clinical infectious disease responsibilities while pregnant, my husband and I agreed that I would not do pediatric and transplant infectious disease rotations until I was past the organogenesis period in the first trimester, the time of greatest risk for most congenitally transmitted infections.

I've been very happy with my career choice and I've never wanted to look seriously at any other area. I am sure I am going to want to do this for the rest of my professional time. I used to love surgical consults, but now I toy with the idea of doing HIV exclusively because it's so interesting. The diseases associated with HIV were once textbook rarities; now they're commonplace. We are developing a sense of how to care for these patients. It is fascinating to be working from the ground up to develop approaches to clinical problems in a field where the approaches didn't exist before.

I would have been happy even if this challenge hadn't come along. There are many interesting questions in infectious diseases. Whether and how a field may change probably should not be a major criterion for picking that field. I suppose you shouldn't go into a specialty because you like only one thing about it; that can put you at risk. If you like many aspects of your specialty, then undoubtedly some of what you like will endure and new areas will attract you. I have never lacked for interesting pursuits. I'm getting old enough that when people ask me what I will do after AIDS, I can say, "I'll retire and write my memoirs" because, unfortunately, I don't think AIDS will go away too soon.

What I do outside of medicine is read. I was an English major in college. As the children have grown, I have begun to read again. I notice that I'm borrowing more nonfiction, whereas at first it was escape reading. The same is happening with my husband, so it may be a stage of life. I just finished a book of excerpts from diaries, letters, and memoirs by pioneer women of the West. We vacation in Montana and I love that part of the country.

I don't think my husband feels that my career has cheated him of time with me. I notice he hasn't tried to divorce me yet. All of our friends and relatives are getting divorced, but we keep saying we'll stick together. I would not have believed 5 years ago that I could talk about retirement, but we're making plans.

I don't think any of our children are giving serious consideration to going into medicine. I would not push them, and I would be pleased only if it were something they really wanted to do. They already feel pressured because I'm a doctor, but I tell them that's not a valid reason to become a doctor without discouraging them from thinking about medicine.

I guess my story sounds all neat and tidy, but there were many junctures where it didn't look like things would work out and when I just about gave up. Probably the worst stress was the trauma of changing my professional direction from tenure track to nontenure track. I felt a little bit like an underachiever because my training program was quite prestigious and many of its alumni have gone on to considerably greater achievements. I was not having success in the project I had chosen; I lacked the imagination and background to know where to turn; and I lacked the commitment to throw myself into it wholeheartedly at the expense of my clinical and teaching activities, a step that might have permitted me to persevere.

I felt like a failure. Then somebody gave me a mug that said, "Success is the repute of honest friends." It was a quote from Emerson (I still have the mug on my desk) and in time I realized that I was happy in the activities that were left to me and that the pride that might have come from proving to the world that I was a worthy member of the succession of achievers from my training laboratory ranked lower than my pleasure in daily life. In fact, I felt lucky to be in a medical school where they would let me stay on and do what I was happy doing and was good at instead of kicking me out because I couldn't do bench research.

Part of what made it such a difficult time was that it wasn't a decision that I made; it all happened to me. I think that was my hardest time professionally. I looked around for other clinical positions and found out that when you're not happy where you are and you want to move, you're not necessarily all that movable. I also learned that in life you can't try to be someone else and do it successfully.

Chapter 13

ONCOLOGY

One of the doctors whom I interviewed for this book described obstetrics as being most often a celebration. If that is so, what, then, is oncology? Viewed from the outside it appears to be a potentially sad and depressing pursuit, but fortunately for the patients who need the services of an oncologist, enough of the physicians who enter the field are able to find sufficient encouragement and comfort in the work to stick with it throughout an entire career.

Dr. Marcia K. Liepman is a staff physician at a large community teaching hospital in Worcester, Massachusetts. She holds an appointment as associate professor of medicine in the school of medicine at the University of Massachusetts Medical Center. Her practice is devoted entirely to the care of people with cancer and blood diseases.

Marcia K. Liepman, M.D., Hematology and Medical Oncology, Private Practice

The perception from outside is that you've got to be tough to take care of oncology patients. For me it turned out that I was comfortable with doing my best to carry a difficult group of patients through the natural history of their disease to death or to cure. Of course it affects me, even now. Sometimes I think I start a mourning process when I meet a patient for the first time.

I'm from the midwest. My mother was college-educated. My father was a butcher who went to night law school in the days when you didn't have to go to college first. And the only doctor I knew was our pediatrician who came to the house to give us penicillin shots. Yet I never considered any career but medicine.

When I was 7, a friend died of leukemia. I was puzzled as to how a perfectly lovely girl could die of this mysterious disease. I guess it stuck in my head that one day I would interact with that disease in some way. I was always better at science and math than English and history, so medicine was a natural for me.

I went to the University of Michigan as a premedical student. I had a scholarship for college and, thank goodness, my parents could afford to put me through medical school. I was lucky enough to finish up with few debts. I went to medical school at Michigan and did my internship, residency, two fellowships, and 5 years of faculty work in Ann Arbor. I married at the end of my junior year in college.

My husband and I met in college. He was a year ahead, and after starting as a physics major he went to medical school. He was going to be a family practitioner, but when Michigan's family practice residency lost federal funding he did a rotating internship, became interested in alcoholism, and ended up in psychiatry. I started medical school with the thought of going into internal medicine or pediatrics. My old interest in leukemia stayed in the background as my orientation toward internal medicine evolved during medical school. I liked all of the clinical rotations, but I related best to adult medicine.

I never considered fields without direct patient contact. The intensity of psychiatry was not my intensity, and the classroom lectures in that field lacked humaneness. Role models were important to me. The first year of medical school was like an extension of college, with 250 students in our class and limited time with faculty. In the third year, our role models were mainly residents, primarily men and fabulous doctors who worked like crazy, took good care of their patients, and were wonderful teachers. The residents did much of the teaching then, but today it's harder for them to do so as their clinical load intensifies.

In my third year I considered surgery but didn't feel I'd be good in the operating room. It wasn't technical ability or the "woman-in-surgery" issue; I simply didn't like the way I felt in the operating room. I realized that as a surgeon, especially during the training years, I could not live the kind of family life that was important to me. I love what surgeons do—they think on their feet and are not afraid to commit—but I could not enjoy doing rounds at 5:30 A.M. Today many of my best friends are surgeons; so it wasn't the people who put me off, it was the lifestyle. Some women have become surgeons and balanced their lives. Many have chosen not to have children or have married and then divorced. The divorce rate in medicine is much higher than in the general population, over 50 percent.

I had reservations about cardiology—I couldn't imagine putting pacemakers in patients in the middle of the night for the rest of my life. Gastroenterology was out because I couldn't see myself doing endoscopy day and night; and pulmonology and endocrinology were out because I didn't enjoy reading their literature. Infectious disease ties you constantly to the hospital. Without any health maintenance organizations (HMOs) around, I figured that I would pursue a career in which I could do some teaching but mostly take care of patients. I didn't think I would be cut out for an academic career or for research. I decided to stay at the university until my husband and I finished training and then find the right setting for taking care of patients.

I don't remember any people or issues that turned me off to a field. When I applied for residency, some program directors made memorable comments like, "What do you think of women in medicine?" What a putdown! At one point I replied, "I can't believe you asked that question." I got no response and was turned down for that residency.

I saw myself as a general internist fighting disease. During my 3-year residency in internal medicine we saw a lot of cancer. The problems were interesting, and when I read about them I could understand what I was reading. I could relate to the people with the disease. The best part of medicine is that you have a fascinating set of problems and you have patients who tell you things they would never tell anybody else.

I had two role models, both women and both superb physicians. One was a hematologist with a family. She was supposedly a part timer but in actuality she worked 60 hours a week. The other was an oncologist who was single. She had been the head of oncology from its inception at Michigan. I felt that like most of the people who trained me, these women demanded excellence. They plus the subject were what eventually led me to hematology–oncology.

First I did a year of hematology because I liked it and wanted to expand my skills as a general internist. I enjoyed the hematology fellowship and signed up for a second year. During that year I did an elective month in medical oncology, a subject that was in its infancy in 1976. You can be in hematology and never deal with cancer, just coagulation, anemia, cytopenia, and the like. But in my fellowship most of what I saw was malignant hematology. Coagulation was a confusing and difficult subject. I loved classical hematology, anemias and the like, and still do.

Then came the elective month of medical oncology. At that time, medical oncology in a university hospital was largely the management of the end-stage disease that followed failure after surgery and radiotherapy. The female oncologist who was my teacher was a fabulous doctor. She knew the natural history of cancers and had a superb understanding of the limitations of diagnostic tests and their role in patient care. I liked being around the patients and tackling the problems you encounter when a 50-year-old patient with pancreatic cancer walks in the door. I also liked taking care of women with breast cancer. The disease fascinated me because it is so common, it affects mainly women, you can really help people with advanced disease, and with hormones the cancers can disappear, at least for a while.

At the end of the hematology fellowship I decided to do an oncology fellowship, but it was June and my mentor had already filled her oncology fellowship. She suggested instead that I run the oncology service at a local VA hospital, and that became my oncology fellowship. I matured quickly as an oncologist and at the end of the year I was a board-certified hemotologist and a board-eligible (ultimately certified) medical oncologist.

Within oncology are subspecialties, depending on where you work. But I had always intended to do a bit of everything. Today I tackle all kinds of cancer and do hematology, even clotting. I doubt that I'm as good in all areas as those oncologists who work in small, limited fields, but I see the patients as they come. Some people come in for cancer phobia though most are referred for a recognized cancer problem. When I hit a stone wall, I make a lot of calls. We get to know our patients well and they usually feel comfortable with us. We commonly send them for second opinions, largely because so much of what we do in oncology is controversial. We also refer patients for special procedures to which we don't have access.

Oncology evolved from hematology because both fields use powerful and potentially toxic drugs, more so than most other specialties. Rheumatology uses a few, pulmonology uses a little methotrexate for asthma, and gastroenterology uses azathioprine and methotrexate for Crohn's disease, but many of the specialists in those fields are uncomfortable when they prescribe the drugs. It's as though it doesn't fit them.

I stayed on at the VA and ran the hematology–oncology section there. After a year, a chief of hematology was appointed and I continued to run the oncology section until I left the midwest. I still saw hematology patients in my clinic. I had trained for both and I knew what I was doing. Some oncologists feel that anybody who thinks they can do both is nuts. Hematology ties in to cardiology and infectious disease through thrombosis and atherosclerosis; viruses also have a lot to do with some of the biology of cancer. Hematology relates to immunology, which creates an intellectual bridge to rheumatology, allergy, and similar areas. Within oncology are medical, surgical, and radiation oncology. Hematologists can be pharmacologists, immunologists, and basic scientists.

The perception from outside is that you've got to be tough to take care of oncology patients. For me it turned out that I was comfortable with doing my best to carry a difficult group of patients through the natural history of their disease to death or cure. Of course it affects me, even now. Sometimes I think I start a mourning process when I meet a patient for the first time. You bond to that person immediately and the two of you become involved in a life-and-death struggle. I do my best for every patient and make sure I know as much as I can about every treatment avenue open to them. Some don't do well and I help them make peace with that. It's not always sad, even when the end is death. No one wants to have cancer, but given what's given, there's a long way you can go with it.

One isn't always looking for the home run. Many of my patients are going to die of their disease but so are cardiologists' patients, for heaven's sake. Some physicians have accosted me with, "Are you going to poison someone today?" Give me a break! That's disrespectful to my patients, to what I do, and to who I am. "Poison" is a terrible word, and the way I hear it used, it's almost as though I'm seen as doing bad things to people on purpose.

I don't have any idea of what it takes to work in my field. Oncologists work hard and get tired, and many of them burn out—because of the schedule, the intensity of the work, and the other goings-on in their lives. I've seen a fair amount of burnout among physicians related to what's happening in their families, such as their kids being alcoholics or taking drugs. It shakes them up because they've put on blinders while trying to do good work. Many doctors in practice, if asked why they went to medical school, would probably answer the same way they did during their admission interview—to help people. There's an idealism to their job, but it can really get crushed by personal problems such as substance abuse, suicidal tendencies, and divorce. Ten to fifteen percent of medical students are substance abusers.

Everybody else predicts that I will burn out in time. I've been at it now for 20 years and my enthusiasm for the work has not changed. There are some oppressive things about the administrative paper work in medicine. We do an awful lot of disability paper work and a lot of arguing with insurance companies about the use of "nonapproved" drugs. Fighting to raise $100,000 for a patient's bone marrow transplant because their insurance company views it as investigational wears you down. If you think things should be done for the good of the patient, it's difficult to keep running into the reality that many decisions in health care have very little to do with the good of the individual patient.

Becoming more expert in my specialty is the major growth that I've experienced as a physician, but it's impossible for me to separate that from what has happened to me as a person. I'm married and have three children from 10 to 20. I started having them during residency and took very little time off. I could manage that because I'm married to a prince and his schedule was compatible with a lot of the child care. He says he didn't have to make any major sacrifices in his career to do that but of course he did. The big dislocations came for both of us when we moved; becoming reacclimated takes time. But we always found good people to whom we could take the children and who understood that we have some late nights.

I have faith that my children have reasonable role models. When they were little, I took care of them when I was home and the babysitter took care of them when I wasn't. As they get older, in some ways it becomes easier and in some ways harder. My husband and I have sort of bumbled through and so far, so good.

Until last year, the 20-year-old said he'd never consider medicine, but he's starting to talk as though maybe it's not such a bad idea. The middle one envisions himself as a highly paid professional athlete. The princess is 10 and just enjoys being happy. My husband and I lucked out with the kids and with our marriage, but it takes a lot of work, especially because we're different types of people.

To get through life, you stumble, have faith, ask questions, and reserve judgment. I was led by the nose. There seems to be more sense of self today, at least among many of the young women. They appear to know where they're going and to be more self-assured than I was. I figured that everything would be okay and didn't ask a lot about how things were done to me or for me. Now, however, I ask a lot about how things are done to or for my patients.

Since I went into oncology the field has changed tremendously. We see patients much earlier in their disease. When I started, most of the patients I saw had failed to respond to all other treatment modalities and we were supposed to give them chemotherapy with a very limited number of drugs. The role of chemotherapy has changed completely. It's viewed as a preventive for recurrence, and in some settings it is given before surgery. Its side effects, formerly intolerable, can be made tolerable, and there are new ways to use it, as there are new forms of treatment such as immunotherapy. Surgeons view their role differently; though they do less surgery, their contribution is still very important. Radiation therapy has become much more than simply "aim and shoot."

I think the oncologist is a more respected member of the team than before. You don't hear quite as much of the "poison" talk. Oncologists and oncology nurses were looked down on in the past. A nurse who worked with me in one of my clinics was ostracized by the other nurses. The thought of handling drugs and dealing with dying people was hard for some of the other nurses. Medical oncologists were viewed as taking the "dregs of humanity" and poisoning them.

My husband and I were in the midwest for a long time and then we needed a change. Our goals in medicine were patient care, teaching, and research, in that order. Our university came out with its goals in 1981 and they were in exactly the reverse order. We started looking for a place with priorities closer to ours and with jobs for both of us. A new medical school seemed reasonable, especially because we weren't ready to cut the ties to academe. The environment near where we lived was not conducive to private practice. The practitioners were struggling in the shadow of the university.

There were places we did not want to live. I had always heard that New England was a nice place to live and raise kids; so in 1982 we found a job for my husband at Brown in Providence, Rhode Island, and one for me at the University of Massachusetts in Worcester. We settled into an old farm halfway between and we're still there. At first I was full time on the UMass faculty and then I went into full-time private practice.

I'm in the hospital around 6:30 A.M. Though I work primarily with the Worcester Memorial Hospital, I visit clinics in small outlying hospitals, which I love, even though it makes for a weird schedule. I go to other hospitals once or twice a week or more to see patients, whom I can follow because of good relationships with their primary care doctors. When I visit clinics only once a week, a nurse fields the calls from sick patients every day so that, through the nurse, they have full access to me. During an emergency, they go to the nearest emergency department. I call ahead to describe the problem and then I call their primary care doctor. Sometimes the patients in other hospitals require things not available in their community so I bring them to Worcester.

I share an office with six doctors: two pure hematologists, one pure oncologist, and the rest hematologist–oncologists. We are independent practitioners and cover for each other. We also teach on the wards of our hospital. I see mostly common cancers: lung, colon, breast. I've never concentrated on one specific condition. I've never worked in a place that had fixed hours. In an HMO, as I understand it, doctors have assigned hours; when they're gone, they're gone. People cover for them at night and the calls stop. That's not the way I have chosen to practice. For me it's preferable to have a relationship with patients that extends beyond daytime hours.

What I love most about medicine is that you can always strive for a higher rung. In choosing a college and medical school you can seek out people who make you strive for more; otherwise, the schools, especially medical school, can turn out to be such a grind as to extinguish your fire. It's hard to know in advance. Talk to people who go there. In choosing a residency, remember that it is by no means an irrevocable decision. You need enough insight to know what turns you on, to understand that first impressions are not always right, and that the worst that can happen is that you may have to go back and train more. In medicine you can do many things. An MD degree can open doors outside of medicine.

When it comes to medicine, I'm idealistic. I think things should be done more for the good of the patient and less for the "good of society." When I helped arrange for a bone marrow transplant on an illegal alien, who paid for it? For my patient faced with a life-threatening disease, it was the best treatment since he had an identical twin. But you and I paid for the transplant and he isn't a citizen. Was it right or wrong? I don't know. I try to understand what's right; I've come to realize that people have complex reasons for what they do. I try to do good and not to do harm.

Chapter 14

DERMATOLOGY

Although some of the physicians represented in this book rejected dermatology because they were uncertain whether it would be broad enough, exciting enough, or demanding enough for them, Dr. Bernhard found it to be all of that and more.

Dr. Jeffrey D. Bernhard is professor of medicine and director of the division of dermatology in the school of medicine at the University of Massachusetts Medical Center in Worcester. He also serves as the medical school's associate dean for admissions.

Jeffrey D. Bernhard, M.D., Dermatology, Academic Medical Center

You also have to trust your intuition. I never sat down with a balance sheet to compare dermatology to endocrinology, for example, in terms of hours on call, financial potential, opportunities for employment, or geographical considerations. A lot depends on what strikes appropriate chords in a person, and people should try to tune in to their inner sense of what they will find stimulating and enjoyable.

The most important factors in my decision to become a dermatologist were good fortune and encounters with inspirational people along the way. I had the good fortune to have enough academic ability to live up to my mother's decision, which seemed to be made when I was in utero, that her son would become a physician. Even so, I like to believe that I wasn't totally programmed. As I reconstruct events, it was positive reinforcement more than pressure.

From early youth I was interested in science—first dinosaurs and then astronomy. For me the closest thing to an early role model was my pediatrician, who would tell me repeatedly that I was going to be a doctor. I went into high school knowing that I was headed toward medical school, and by my freshman year of college I knew that I would choose dermatology.

I had a science teacher in my freshman year of high school who pointed me to Harvard. The idea was completely out of kilter with my folks' economic circumstances; neither of them had completed college. The same teacher also directed me to a National Science Foundation summer program at Roswell Park Memorial Institute in Buffalo, which is where I grew up. High school kids came here to work in the lab with Roswell Park scientists during the summer. It was wonderful—the kids came from all over the country and were paid $10 a week. My first summer I was assigned to an immunohematologist who was studying the effect of laser radiation on serum proteins and antibodies.

For about 6 weeks, I detected no effects; so, to check more thoroughly, I stayed one night and repeated the assay every hour. At midnight, I went to the hospital lobby to buy a soda and ran into the chief of dermatology, a wild, wonderful workaholic who came in whenever he felt like it. He invited me to his office to talk about my work; he asked me why lasers weren't used to treat skin tumors. I learned later that he was doing research on the question. I answered, "Because we're concerned that the radiation might disperse tumor cells." He said I was right and invited me to work in his lab the following summer, which I did and had a fantastic time. He was inspirational and very enthusiastic about dermatology. "If you want to solve the cancer problem," he said, "what better field than dermatology where you can see the tumors? Besides, academic medicine is a difficult world; so another benefit of dermatology is that if a dean ever gives you a hard time, you can just walk out and open up a private practice."

If I hadn't met him, I'm positive I would have been an endocrinologist. There surely wasn't much encouragement to go into dermatology. Except for the dermatologists, my classmates and teachers in medical school did not consider dermatology a premier specialty. I would like to believe that when I took the dermatology rotation I would have realized that I was suited to the field.

I can remember things that I see, and visual memory is a big part of dermatology. With this ability, I suppose that I could have gone into pathology. During medical school and my initial clinical training, I also came to realize that the working conditions in dermatology are attractive. As a way of life, it's more controllable than many other specialties. You can manage your own time, control what you do, and set limits, at least with regard to getting up in the middle of the night and coming in on weekends.

By going on rounds with the dermatology chief at Roswell Park I learned that dermatology is intriguing and fun. Furthermore, because I saw patients with mycosis fungoides and malignant melanoma, it never occurred to me that there was anything trivial about the field. He cared for very sick people, some of whom were dying, and made a real difference. He developed the use of topical 5-fluorouracil for actinic keratoses and was one of the early people in tumor immunology. In short, the skin was a perfect venue for scientific investigation. Later, during medical school, the clinical acumen and great enthusiasm of the professors of dermatology greatly enhanced my enchantment with the skin. They had the capacity to make the problems and questions in dermatology as enthralling as those in any other field of biology and medicine.

After medical school, my internship was in general medicine and at one point I thought of doing 3 years of medicine. I met people who loved their work and were excited about it. I had several excellent experiences with endocrinologists, but eventually dermatology won out.

Today it is helpful for a student to decide about dermatology during the fourth year of medical school so he or she can apply for a position that will become available in July of the year after internship. For people who want to take an additional 2 years of medicine before their dermatology training, many programs encourage that. The problem, though, is that federal regulations prohibit Medicare from reimbursing hospitals for doctors in a second residency past the fifth year of total training, and the dermatology residency is a 3-year program. This makes it difficult to fund the sixth year of training.

I have no regrets about my choice of dermatology. Instead of being constricting, knowing early on what I wanted to do had a liberating effect. To me it meant that I didn't have to expend any energy wondering about other possibilities and could attach things to a framework that I had in my mind. In picking a residency, I believed that the best available program was located in Boston, right across town, and I was lucky enough to be admitted. A student should be on the alert for the most attractive program and place himself or herself in a position where he or she can be exposed to a variety of experiences. There is something unique and wonderful about academic environments in which people are trying to advance the frontiers of knowledge. That certainly clicked for me.

You also have to trust your intuition. I never sat down with a balance sheet to compare dermatology to endocrinology, for example, in terms of hours on call, financial potential, opportunities for employment, or geographical considerations. A lot depends on what strikes appropriate chords in a person, and people should try to tune in to their inner sense of what they will find stimulating and enjoyable.

My decision to enter academic medicine as opposed to private practice was based on the purely selfish attraction of having an opportunity to be excited every day at work, to be stimulated by new problems and questions, and to learn something new every day. I thought I could find these only in an academic environment. Also, I wanted a situation whereby I was not just working to live but living to work. One of the amusing and ironic things about the notion of dermatology not controlling my life is that it doesn't mean I work any less; it simply means that maybe I have a little more control over the way I divide up the 60 or 80 hours a week that I spend working. It doesn't mean that I'm not plugging away on nights and weekends.

After I trained in dermatology, I spent an extra year as a dermatology clinical and research fellow working in photobiology. This was a lucky opportunity because the field had been opened up by my mentors and I was in on the excitement of breaking new ground and helping many people through new treatments and technologies.

During that year, I began to understand what kind of academician I wanted to be—a clinician. I did not want to do basic bench research. I felt that I could not combine laboratory research with patient care and clinical investigation and be good at both. I hoped to investigate clinical problems and develop expertise at the leading edge of clinical practice. I moved here in 1983, and 3 years later the person who recruited me went into private practice, so I became director of the division. In addition to all the fun aspects of the art and science of practicing dermatology, I have had the satisfaction of building a little division of dermatology.

One of the wonderful things about my work is that I interact with a variety of people on a daily basis. Every day is different, although there are some consistencies from week to week in what I do: I see patients for three clinical sessions a week and I work on medical school admissions one day a week. I do the latter because I care about the institution and its students.

In the clinic I interact with students and medical residents on a regular basis. For one week in the school curriculum (a grossly inadequate time) we teach second-year students dermatology. I administer our dermatology division, where I work with nurses, secretaries, and other staff, and am involved in human relations problem solving. In addition, I serve on editorial boards of several dermatology journals and have written a book about itching.

I try to think of clinical questions that I can answer and write about them. One thing I cherish most is thinking and writing. Time for that is hardest to come by and easily stolen away by the pressure of other things; this activity takes time away from the family. Although it's a struggle to achieve balance, right now I'm very pleased with they way things are and don't foresee becoming dissatisfied. We're still building. For example, we're going to start a dermatology residency here in July. I can imagine some pressure to decrease my work with patients. If my patient care time falls too low, though, I know I'll begin to feel that I am no longer a doctor.

Students should keep an open mind and remain individualistic. They should look for opportunities to interact with exciting individual faculty members. They shouldn't be shy about knocking on a lecturer's door and saying, "I enjoyed your talk. The material was exciting. May I work in your lab and follow you on rounds?" Faculty members appreciate that and the rewards for the students are priceless. A poet once said, "Follow your bliss." Students should do that.

Chapter 15

OPHTHALMOLOGY

Although today the application process for entering ophthalmology pressures medical students to make a decision about entering the field almost during the third year of medical school, Dr. Harris didn't choose his direction until he had completed a rotating internship and had decided on internal medicine. His story tells about that decision, about an enduring interest in the economic and organizational aspects of medicine, and about life in an HMO.

Dr. William K. Harris is a long-term member of the Department of Ophthalmology at Kaiser Permanente, Northwest Region, in Portland, Oregon.

William K. Harris, M.D., Ophthalmology,
Health Maintenance Organization

The opportunity to make valuable improvements in a person's vision quickly is a great reward. . . . I've maintained my enthusiasm for ophthalmology largely because it has evolved in many interesting directions over these years.

My decision to become a doctor evolved over time. As a child in a small community in West Virginia, I regarded our two practicing physicians as materialistic and pompous. Once, when I was seen for a serious eye injury by an ophthalmologist 25 miles away, he told my father in my presence that I would lose my eye. Today the eye is fine, but his callous behavior stayed with me for years and delayed my entry into medicine. I studied engineering at West Virginia University and planned to attend law school, but in my senior year I realized that my negative ideas about doctors were not so valid and, for a mixture of reasons I applied to medical school.

Above and beyond providing status and a satisfactory income, medicine appeared interesting and useful to society. I became concerned with medical economics and, after reading and writing about it, I concluded that the way Americans paid for medical care was crazy. For me, the reasonable way to give medical care was to become a doctor. I wanted to avoid being so preoccupied with personal economic gain that I lost sight of what makes life worthwhile; I have pursued my interest in the economics of medical care ever since.

I took the medical school prerequisites and entered West Virginia's 2-year, state medical school. For my third- and fourth-year clinical experiences I transferred to the University of Pennsylvania where I was attracted to the scientific sophistication of internal medicine. I got to know an exciting city, met students from all over the country, worked in several hospitals, and met the woman who would become my wife.

The clerkships confirmed my inclination toward internal medicine. I didn't consider surgery because I was more comfortable with internists' personalities. Surgeons seemed sensitive to appearances and uncomfortable to be around or to know as friends. I don't know why I didn't turn to pediatrics, and my experience with psychiatry was a combination of distrust and partial understanding. As for radiology and pathology, the distance from the patient was too great.

I spent my third-year summer elective looking at a New York City organization called "H.I.P." for Health Insurance Plan. It was an early version of "HMO" and "managed care." In the 1950s there was great hope that society would structure its medical care through a broad insurance base in a prepaid comprehensive health care program. I was attracted by the concept that everyone paid to maintain the system and used it freely, but only as needed.

For that to work, however, physicians must play the crucial role of distributing care according to need, and we haven't been successful at that. We still distribute medical care according to the patient's appetite. Practitioners become stressed trying to differentiate between pleasing patients and doing what is appropriate within the bounds of available resources. I'm talking about rationing health care, where the primary care doctor is the gatekeeper who gives to this patient and holds back from that one, and who tries to clarify for patients what is useful for them as opposed to doing whatever they want. That is not easy. Decisions such as whether a 70-year-old man should have a heart transplant cannot be left solely to the physician, but they shouldn't be made arbitrarily.

My H.I.P. experience left me wanting to explore such ideas. The only opportunities were with Kaiser in the west and H.I.P. in the east. Because I wanted to keep my training broad and because I was curious about the west coast, I ended up in a rotating internship at the King County Hospital, now called Harborview, in Seattle. It was a city hospital just beginning a relationship with the nearby medical school. My program was separate from the school's but it was the highlight of my training years. We rotated through the emergency room, obstetrics and gynecology, general surgery, pediatrics, medicine, and neurology. We saw surgical subspecialties but not much otolaryngology (ENT) or ophthalmology.

I had met my wife-to-be in Philadelphia when she was a journalist. Five years later she joined me in Seattle where we were married in the summer after my internship. During that year I took my first training in internal medicine by working with a new King County home health care program. Then, in the early 1960s, I joined the army for 2 years to fulfill a deferred military obligation.

I entered the army interested in internal medicine and left it committed to ophthalmology. For 2 years I was assigned near Pisa, Italy, to do general practice in a 60-bed general hospital for American forces and dependents attached to NATO. Most of the medical work was done by me and another generalist—neither of us had any specialty training in internal medicine.

Several factors led me to ophthalmology. One was discovering how concerned my patients were about their eyes. I would focus on someone's poor cardiopulmonary function but the patient would be interested only in vision problems. I spent time with an Italian ophthalmologist who made occasional visits to our hospital. My medical school roommate wrote to tell me why he had switched from pediatrics to ophthalmology, and eventually I decided to do the same.

I found a residency by sheer luck. The doctors' draft for the Vietnam War had depleted my ex-roommate's residency program at the Wills Eye Hospital in Philadelphia; just as I was leaving the army, a slot opened up there. When my friend told me about it, I applied and was accepted.

I was attracted especially to the surgical aspect of ophthalmology because I enjoy the precise work involved in the craft. The opportunity to make valuable improvements in a person's vision quickly is a great reward. Probably I could have moved into general surgery, ENT, or orthopedics with equal enthusiasm. It's different today. Students must decide on ophthalmology very early to make training arrangements, or they must delay for several years while searching for a vacant residency slot. I don't see how a second-year medical student can know enough to decide on ophthalmology unless an interest stems from earlier direct experience. One should have a prior exposure to an ophthalmologist's office and operating room practice. It is no longer necessary in ophthalmology to be especially skillful at the mechanics or the surgical aspects because now there are opportunities in ophthalmic subspecialties that do not emphasize surgery.

The discipline roughly divides into medical and surgical portions. Some practitioners do more surgery, some limit their surgery to the use of lasers, and some practice neuroophthalmology and do almost no surgery at all. Eye surgery is a good choice for a person skilled in the use of hand tools and automated equipment, one who is stimulated, not stressed, by high stakes precision work.

My residency training took 3 years. I worked hard, learned a lot, and felt right about being in ophthalmology. When I finished, I wanted to be broad-based and work in an HMO, preferably in the Pacific Northwest where we liked the weather and outdoor activities. I went to Kaiser Permanente in Portland, where I've been in general ophthalmology ever since. In 1970, it was a reasonably small HMO. Today it is much larger. After more than 20 years here, I feel that the social and economic factors are more prominent in a doctor's life back east. Here society is freer and more open, although Oregon has turned out to be much less populist than we expected.

Life in an HMO has been especially rewarding. I am a member of a small group of interdependent-minded ophthalmologists whom I have liked and respected for years. Their humaneness and technical ability exceeds what I could have found otherwise. We don't always get along perfectly, but part of the excitement arises from differences in opinions and values. Most of our conflicts are purposeful.

A doctor in an HMO does not need to pay as much attention to the business aspects of the office as does the physician–owner of a practice. More caring medicine can be provided in an HMO because of fewer economic constraints. I am suspicious of the current concern about medicine's "loss of humanity." I sense that much of the apparent caring in the past stemmed more from the doctor caring about the patient socially rather than clinically. Being sweet to people may not help a patient's health. Indeed, if it makes the patient more dependent on the doctor, it may be counterproductive. The important thing is that two people work together to identify and solve or manage a problem that both consider important. This can be preserved nicely in the HMO setting. I think that in this country today the Kaiser pattern is the most rational approach available.

I am concerned that over the years the Kaiser staff may not have maintained the same idealism that was present at the start. I miss that fervor, but its decline is understandable because we are no longer viewed as an illegitimate system and no longer need to defend our approach. We'll never restore the initial level of excitement, but I hope the doctors in our group share my view that what we're doing is the country's main defense against developing a national program that cannot provide purposeful medical care at an appropriate cost.

Our free time is truly free because colleagues cover for us. I take my vacations confident that my patients will receive good care. It's financially easier for me to take time to study and go to professional meetings than it is for someone in an individual practice. People say that HMO physicians regard their jobs as nine-to-five assignments and are not as able or as dedicated as in other settings. That is not so in our HMO. In dollar terms my lifetime income here probably will be about 60 percent of what it might have been, but the practice could not have been as rich and rewarding.

I'm on a salary, a portion of which is at risk within our physician corporation, but due to the system's size, income fluctuations are small. We physicians elect a board of directors to make decisions for our organization. It contracts annually to care for the Kaiser patients. When I joined Kaiser Permanente, it comprised 80–100 doctors; now there are over 300.

Deciding how much to pay doctors is frustrating. A doctor's responsibility should be to efficiently detect and then solve or manage the medical problems in a population of people. The number of patients I see in a day is of interest, but the crucial question is what kind of progress my interventions make during the day in identifying and dealing with the eye problems of the 370,000 enrolled people. If half of my office time involves seeing people who do not have a problem and who are not any better off for having seen me, then that should not be counted as a positive effort. There will inevitably be lots of that, but simply doing that isn't vital and doesn't deserve a fee. To the extent that our program looks only at the work we do and gives each unit of work a dollar value, as in a fee-for-service arrangement, I think it misses the boat. Merely "doing" is not the critical role. Rather, it is doing what is pertinent that counts.

An unnecessary or frivolous visit to the doctor may seem okay to the patient but it's bad for society because we all have to pay the bill and the patient is misled about the value of the visit. Most public education about medical problems rests heavily on mystifying illness and aggrandizing the medical industry. For example, the idea that the asymptomatic human eye should be checked once a year for maladies that need early attention is not useful and generates fear. The eye is honest and will speak up. Similarly, the routine general physical exam probably is not a useful practice.

Today's society doesn't know what it wants in the way of care for illness and injury, doesn't know how to find out, doesn't have the money to pay for what is being consumed now, and is without the means to decide what is worth buying. If you don't know what you want and you don't know when you've got it, you're in no position to decide if the price is right. We have an immense educational challenge.

In our group we try to communicate to our patients, when appropriate, that annual eye exams aren't useful because nothing can happen during the next 5 years that their eyes won't tell them about. We should teach our patients what conditions we know to be genuine risks and worth medical encounters and help them to assess when to seek an examination. Unfortunately, patients sometimes seem to believe that we are just trying to cut back on expenses because our system is prepaid. A key issue today in health care is the disparity between the money patients are willing to pay for services and their appetite for services, many of questionable value, that cost far more.

I think it is important for primary care doctors to deal with eye-related complaints. It is so unnecessary that a patient with a small foreign object trapped under the upper lid drive many miles to see an ophthalmologist when the problem could be taken care of at home or at a nearby medical facility. We work with primary care practitioners to help them overcome their fear of the eye, manage problems when they are able, and refer appropriately.

Had I been in a private group, I probably would not have pursued this concern about the health care of the greater society. I would have had to build a new practice instead of starting out with a full one. The use of paraprofessionals is a fundamental approach of the Kaiser system. We've been criticized for this, but unjustly. Nurse practitioners and physicians' assistants are remarkably caring and skillful. Optometrists do the refractions and eye health exams in our department, and they do a superb job. The use of physician extenders is a wonderful concept.

I have no comprehensive solutions to the problems of health care. Organizing it in a system offers advantages only up to a certain size and only as long as discussion and values can influence behavior. In time, our Kaiser system in Oregon will provide enough patient education so our subscribers' understanding and our physicians' activities will be in harmony and we will be providing what people want and consider reasonable to pay for. We can't do that as a nation because it requires individuals to recognize that they belong to a group of people, all of whom invest in the same health insurance complex and on whom it is incumbent to use the coverage in a manner that makes the system sustainable.

Patients and the medical industry need to be sensitive to interdependencies, but these days "interdependence" is seldom understood and "independence" is worshipped. People want their own medical concerns seen to conveniently and immediately and without regard for interdependence. It would be silly to make national decisions right now on issues that require an appreciation of interdependence for success. Our public is not ready to listen. Until we cooperate for the common good, socializing medicine over a wide geographic area will not work. An excellent alternative lies in multiple, varied, smaller organizations like ours with a single national payer.

Serving indigent people requires tax money. The 1994 Oregon plan is very encouraging. About 15 years ago I had hoped that we would establish a statewide blue-ribbon lay legislative committee to evaluate diagnostic and therapeutic activities in medicine, decide their financial worth to us as individuals, buy this for the medically indigent, and require that all health insurers also offer this basic package to the general public. The Oregon plan may cause this to occur.

To support the introduction of new and not yet fully evaluated modalities of care, society will have to pay for that care as though it were worthwhile, even before it becomes so. We have to distinguish those things that are investigational from those that are highly useful but simply require a great deal of volume to permit the cost savings. The entire nation had better do this instead of forcing medical schools and their research and training programs into the crazy position of trying to use insurance money to pay for research. As for new clinical procedures, Oregon's approach will permit their development, but at a slower pace. There will be fewer false starts and less unnecessary morbidity.

Ophthalmology is very different from when I started because now we can do many more useful things. This is both gratifying and frustrating since not every patient benefits from the new treatments. Laser photocoagulation of the retina prevents or minimizes complications of diabetic retinopathy statistically for a group of patients, but some patients would do just as well without it. Because we don't make unsuccessful patients much worse, we offer the treatment to all patients in order to reach the ones who can be helped.

We can do remarkably more to rehabilitate the cataract-limited eye than we could 20 years ago when cataract removal required the patient to spend 5 days in the hospital and optical correction required thick spectacles or contact lenses. In elderly patients the hospital stay led to such serious complications as deterioration of mental status and pulmonary embolism, and afterward there was considerable morbidity to being without a lens in the eye. Today, because the patient is hardly in the hospital and placement of a plastic lens makes rehabilitation so remarkably effective, a cataract can be removed without causing much trouble. We can restore vision to so nearly fully functional that there is virtually no interruption of the patient's essential life activities.

Incorporation of the microscope in eye surgery has made it possible to see what we are doing. Major clinical challenges include managing macular degeneration, caring for the eyes of diabetic people, and treating glaucoma. We still have numerous patients who lose their reading vision in later years. Glaucoma is an example of improved treatment with continuing challenge. It is widespread and becoming more of a problem as we live longer. It is an inexorable, progressive chronic illness that seldom if ever stops at a specific stage unless we intervene. Management of glaucoma is cumbersome and has only qualified success. Some patients receive the best treatment available and still lose vision. The medicines have become much less morbid and the drops are remarkably more effective than they were 20 years ago. Surgery for glaucoma continues to improve.

I've maintained my enthusiasm for ophthalmology largely because it has evolved in many interesting directions over these years. Almost one quarter of my work time is spent doing surgery. In recent years my practice has shifted from broad general ophthalmology (retinal surgery, muscle surgery for children or adults with deviating eyes, glaucoma surgery, and cataract surgery) to a marked increase in cataract surgery. The repair of retinal detachment that many of us did as general ophthalmologists 20 years ago is now mainly done by people specialized in treatment of the retina.

As a generalist, my practice involves managing people with cataracts, glaucoma, cross-eyes, lid trouble (such as lids hanging too low), inflammatory conditions and periocular cancers of the skin. There is now fellowship training in ophthalmologic plastic surgery, in which the practice is limited to correcting lid deformities, removing lid tumors, and doing surgery of the orbit to excise orbital tumors. Even surgery for corneal grafting became specialized 20 years ago. I do neuroophthalmology unless the case is an unusual one and I am uncertain about the diagnosis or unfamiliar with the treatment. Inherited diseases are a small and growing part of my practice. Because some age-related macular degeneration can be effectively treated by laser, much of our time is spent finding the people who have a treatable form and stage of the condition.

A large segment of our work is with ambulatory patients. Hospital admissions are almost limited to ocular injuries associated with other trauma that requires the hospitalization. This change toward ambulatory care in contrast to hospitalizing the whole body to take care of the eye represents a delightful improvement.

I'm so far away from residency training that I can say little about how a second-year medical student should go about deciding to become an ophthalmologist and compete for a training position. It looks like a dreadful encumbrance to the person who's trying to plan his or her life. All training programs include a general ophthalmology residency before entering into a subspecialty of the eye. There are no internships in ophthalmology, and people who go into ophthalmology must serve in an internship in some other realm first. I think it would be best if it were a general experience. The established subspecialties in ophthalmology now include pediatrics, cornea (which often relates to cataract), glaucoma, vitreoretinal, plastic, and neuroophthalmology.

When going into medicine it is important to plan as far into the future as practical. The purpose is not to follow the plan literally but to provide oneself with the tranquility to respond to change with a clear mind and an unburdened heart. None of us can make wisest choices until the circumstances actually present. Although medicine has its imperfections, it provides a stellar career. Being a physician allows one to participate in society's attempts to shape things in a form that improves our lives.

Chapter 16

UROLOGY

Dr. Menon's professional journey took him from India to the United States and from neurosurgery to cardiac surgery to urologic surgery. All along he had his sights fixed on a position in academic medicine.

Dr. Mani Menon is professor of surgery and physiology and chairman of the Division of Urologic and Transplantation Surgery in the Department of Surgery of the school of medicine at the University of Massachusetts Medical Center in Worcester.

Mani Menon, M.D., Urology, Academic Medical Center

I don't know exactly how a student in the second or third year of medical school can make the decision to enter urology, but I do believe that most of the students who rotate on urology would be happy working in the field.

I went to medical school in India where career decisions are mostly decided for you. After 1 or 2 years of college, you can go to professional school for medicine or engineering or you can first get an undergraduate degree. Everyone is eligible to apply, so if you are among the top 100, or top 2 percent, of the applicants, you get into medical school.

When I was 16, my mother suggested that I apply for both engineering and medicine and pick one later. I preferred engineering. However, my medical school interview preceded my engineering school interview and I accepted a medical school position despite having thought that I would be an engineer since my strengths were in mathematics, physics, and chemistry. I might have become an engineer and loved it, but I'm happy with what I'm doing. I have no regrets. Winston Churchill said that the weakness of second guessing is that you never know what would have happened if you had gone with your second guess.

Our medical school was one of the two national ones. We had 75 students in our class, 65 of them college valedictorians, and the final exams were so tough that only 12 of us graduated without having to repeat a year. The intellectual students were expected to go into internal medicine or a subspecialty; students who were good with their hands into surgery or a subspecialty; and students who were neither into orthopedics. Our chairman of orthopedic surgery was very smart and gifted with his hands, which gave the lie to that particular notion.

Because I graduated close to the top of my class, my professors advised internal medicine. Besides, I wasn't good at things like breaking up a watch and putting it back together. Logic seemed to dictate internal medicine, so it was surprising that I chose surgery.

I became interested in surgery during my second year. We spent 18 months in gross anatomy, physiology, and biochemistry. I didn't like dissecting cadavers, but I learned that there is a beautiful logic in the way the human body is constructed. I also liked the fact that I could mentally visualize a structure and then actually dissect it out. That turned me on to surgery.

After finishing medical school at age 20, I did 3 years of general surgery in India, aiming to be a brain surgeon because I felt that neurosurgery was the most intellectual branch of surgery. In India all surgeons train for 3 years and get a masters degree in general surgery. Then they can subspecialize. After my general surgery training, I came to this country planning to train in neurosurgery and return to India. When I came here, they gave me credit for attending medical school in India, but they didn't credit any of my postgraduate training, so I had to start over again—as a surgical intern in a community hospital. Then I applied to and was rejected by every neurosurgical program in the country. Most of them didn't even reply, I guess because I was a foreign medical graduate.

On the neurosurgery rotation during my internship, I found that neurosurgery as practiced in a community hospital is very different from that in India. India has one neurosurgeon for maybe 10 million people. There neurosurgeons operate on the brain almost exclusively, removing many benign tumors and saving lives. In this country, much of the neurosurgery I saw was back surgery. As for the few brain tumors and aneurysms that we did operate on, the results were not always good because the vast majority of the tumors were malignant, which was disheartening.

Thinking ahead about my medical career, I wanted an academic position. Private practice never crossed my mind. My medical school was very academic. In most Indian medical schools the faculty were what we call here "clinical faculty," generating almost all of their income from private practice. As a pilot project, the federal Indian government had set up two national medical schools with full-time faculty, and ours was one. My exposure there led me to feel that you could be much more altruistic if you were not distracted by financial matters. I enjoyed teaching and working with the other residents, and I wanted the immediate gratification of playing a critical role in helping the patient.

During my neurosurgery rotation, I was exposed to a role model who was so far from ideal that, given my experience with the residency applications, my disenchantment with the nature of the problems I saw in practice here, and my preceptor's example, I was thoroughly soured on the field. My next rotation was urology, and there I met a far superior role model.

He was a bright, vigorous, and superbly talented surgeon. Instead of making me feel like an intruder, as had occurred in neurosurgery, he made me feel like the greatest thing since sliced bread. I went on to the urology service with an open mind and a genuine interest in exploring all fields. In contrast, the American house officers had pretty much decided before internship what they were going to do. And so those already committed to something else—otolaryngology, for example—would view the urology rotation as merely biding time and not deserving of a great deal of effort.

I threw myself into urology heart and soul. Consequently, I was given preferential treatment and did many interesting procedures. In particular, there was a lot of stone surgery that inspired my fascination with renal stones and with urology as a discipline. A patient would come in with excruciating pain and a big kidney stone, you would do a 40-minute operation, and the patient would be pain-free. In addition, you could search for an explanation of why the kidney stones formed in the first place. You operated on patients with cancer who were not terminally ill. You saw patients with obstructive uropathy who couldn't urinate and you could relieve them with endoscopic surgery. You also did diagnostic work. You didn't just explore patients to try to find out what was wrong, as happened in a lot of general surgery (at least in the era before CAT scans). Because of the sophistication of the radiologic techniques, you knew in advance that a patient had a stone or a transitional cell carcinoma, and I liked that.

In medical school I did not take to the fields removed from contact with patients; for example, pathology was never a possibility. I could never diagnose whether something was benign or malignant by looking at a slide. Our dean was a distinguished pathologist who had a profound influence on me, yet I never thought of going into his discipline.

It's wrong to make decisions early on. During medical school you can make a good decision about the broad field—internist, surgeon, pediatrician, or nonclinician such as anatomist, pathologist, or radiologist. you can concentrate on that when you rotate on the specialties during the third year of medical school, but that is not the time to decide whether you are going to be a gastroenterologist or cardiologist. In a way, medicine and the medical specialties offer students a better pathway for making that sort of decision because every medical specialist first needs to become a general internist.

The surgical specialties present a real problem because you might decide early on to go into ophthalmology and find that you dislike it. The old rotating internship that vanished in the 1970s was very helpful. You spent 3 months in medicine, 3 in surgery, 3 in pediatrics, and 3 in one nonclinical specialty. Then, at the end of the year, you decided what you wanted to be.

In April of my internship year I decided that I liked urology, but I had already committed myself to the general surgery track and had accepted a second-year slot in it. Besides, the people who were going into urology had been picked 2 years earlier, and there was no way that I could rationally hope to get into a urology program.

Nowadays to train in urology you need 2 years of general surgery first, but the urology residents are picked as fourth-year medical students. Usually the urology programs prefer to have you do general surgery at their institutions so they can get to know you.

I found a place in urology by a stroke of luck. About the time that

I decided to go into urology, I started my rotation in cardiac surgery. I worked with a cardiac surgeon who was a former academic. A fine human being, he was one of the first pediatric cardiac surgeons in the country. He had missed out on a major university chair in that field and had entered private practice.

I approached cardiac surgery just as I had approached neurosurgery and urology; that is, by learning a lot and doing my best even though I had no intention of becoming a heart surgeon. Because my wife was visiting her family in India and I had not yet made friends in America, I took call at the hospital, which was across the street from where we lived, just about all of the time. I made rounds on my patients at midnight 7 nights a week as did the man who was to become my mentor. That's how we came to know each other. Although I explained to him that I was making rounds because I had nothing better to do, he thought I had a burning interest in his field. In time, he strongly encouraged me to become a cardiac surgeon.

During that time, he was doing mainly coronary artery bypass surgery, like most other heart surgeons. I wanted much more variety and told him that I hoped to become a urologist. As others had, he told me that I was too talented and smart to be a urologist. He proposed to find me a spot in cardiac surgery, set up a program for me, and eventually take me into a handsome private practice with him.

I held out for urology and finally he said that if I really meant it, there was only one person with whom I should train, a man who had once been his intern and who was good enough to have become a heart surgeon but had become a urologist instead. His friend was about to take over the chairmanship of a department in a major university. "I'll call him," he said, "and see whether he will give you a job."

I thought, "Oh sure, this heart surgeon in private practice will call up the chairman, and he will give me a spot in urology when there aren't any to be had because of the 2-years-in-advance system." Two or 3 days later, he came by and said it was all set, but there was a small catch. I thought, "Here it comes." There were no funds to pay me.

I said that I didn't see how I could work without any salary, but he told me not to worry. He had informed the dean of the medical school that he would pay my salary for a year. When I said I couldn't take his money, he replied, "If you don't you will insult me. It's not a great deal of money for me and I'm interested in helping people. That's why I became a doctor. The way to help you is to get you into that program. If you are so foolish as to want to be a urologist, then you must become an excellent one." And that's how I entered urology. My mentor is a phenomenal person and we've remained friends to this day.

It's interesting to think about physicians' attitudes toward the different fields of medicine. By and large, we regard our own specialty as the only good one. The cardiac surgeon felt that urology was terrible, but the cardiologist with whom I worked said, "You don't want to go into cardiac surgery! We cardiologists make the diagnosis. The surgeons just saw open the chest and sew a couple of things together. Any fool can do that. What's important is making that diagnosis and telling the surgeons what they need to do." The neurosurgeon felt that what he was doing was most important, but the neurologist felt that neurosurgeons were just a bunch of hacks and that diagnoses had to be made for them. Maybe to survive we need to tell ourselves that only our work is important. In rotating from one specialty to another, I found that I could be happy in most of them.

But there were some I didn't enjoy, orthopedics for example. I believe this was because I just did not like the chairman of orthopedics at my medical school. It is unfortunate that we make decisions on such a flimsy basis because orthopedics is a fine field. Many of my close friends went into orthopedics, and I respect them and what they do. Although I felt I wouldn't enjoy pathology, I would have been happy doing radiology.

I don't know exactly how a student in the second or third year of medical school can make the decision to enter urology, but I do believe that most of the students who rotate on urology would be happy working in the field. Part of the reason is that we are not under constant severe pressure, not always making life-and-death decisions, and we see tangible benefit from what we do for our patients. That improves a physician's quality of life.

A patient can be made miserable by a kidney stone, but he isn't going to die as a result of it. You can be in urinary retention and feel as though you are going to die, but you won't. You can have great patient satisfaction with results of your work because you can take care of their problems fairly expeditiously. It's a specialty that is fairly narrow, so you don't feel that you're always missing something in the literature, and you can feel confident that you really know what you're doing. Emergencies are infrequent because you can anticipate things and do a high percentage of elective surgery. I think that the people who go into urology are attracted to these attributes of the field. There used to be barriers to women in our field, but things are evolving and now we are looking for women. There still aren't many; maybe 100 out of the 7000 urologists are women.

In balancing your life as a physician, everything has to give a little. As an academic urologist I don't spend as much time with my patients as I would if I were simply doing patient care. I'm not as good a researcher as I would be if I were just doing research. I'm not as good an administrator as I would be if all I were doing was administration. And I'm not probably as good a father as I might be if I were not a doctor. You try to balance it all as best you can.

I'm happy with the way things have worked out for me, but I have misgivings too. I'm human and I sometimes wonder how different it would have been if I had become a heart surgeon. Two changes have happened in urology that make me less enthusiastic than I was when I started. Then what I enjoyed the most was the surgery of stones and taking care of patients with stone problems. But during the last 5 years, lithotripsy has changed that and I've been put out of business. I spent 9 years developing an operation for stone disease that would minimize morbidity but it isn't nearly as good as lithotripsy. Yet I was one of the people who helped to develop lithotripsy. It's best for the patients, but it is pretty boring. If I were going into urology now, I might think twice because of that.

The field you choose at the start of your career can change. Urology has become much more medical. And yet when I entered it, I liked urology because of its combination of medicine and surgery. I wouldn't want to be in the operating room every single day, as I would be if I were a heart surgeon or a plastic surgeon. I enjoy making a diagnosis and treating. When I started, urology was 75 percent surgical and 25 percent medical. Now it's closer to 40 percent surgical and 60 percent medical. I never wanted to be that much of an internist.

Still, I think I will stay with it. I don't see more attractive pathways. The logical thing would be administration, but what I enjoy most is looking after patients and being in the operating room.

Chapter 17

ORTHOPEDIC SURGERY

This story shows that a strong and active interest in the sociological underpinnings of medicine is compatible with a career choice that emphasizes the technical aspects. Since the story is only at its midpoint, it may yet come full circle.

Dr. Gerald G. Steinberg is professor of orthopedic surgery and vice chairman in the Department of Orthopedics and Physical Rehabilitation in the medical school of the University of Massachusetts Medical Center in Worcester. Recently, he was appointed chief medical officer (chief of staff) of the medical center.

Gerald G. Steinberg, M.D., Orthopedic Surgery, Academic Medical Center

Even though it may sound as though I was on a focused pathway when I made my decision, my career could have gone in a different direction if I had found a mentor in general surgery, ophthalmology, or another area. . . . Taking the attitude that you will bloom wherever you are planted rather than searching for the ideal plot of soil probably brings greater success and comfort.

As far back as age 6, medicine was what I wanted to pursue. Doctors seemed important, powerful, and helping, and I wanted to be like them. In our family a child who wanted to be a doctor gained smiles and favorable comments. There were times later on, particularly after I finished my training, when I questioned my decision, and even now, I often think about what else I could have done. But it is mostly "what-if" musing about other talents that remain undeveloped. In fact I'm quite happy.

I always enjoyed the sciences and majored in biology in college. At age 15, I worked in a drugstore after school and on weekends. Within his abilities the pharmacist taught me which medication was appropriate for which symptoms and he enhanced my understanding of what sick people need and how people in different economic circumstances deal with illness. All of this reinforced my feelings that I might be a good physician.

In medical school I became active in the Student Health Organization, a group that developed in the late 1960s. Our main issues were related to health care: access, financing, socioeconomic, and demographic aspects of provision of services, community organizational issues, and the relation of health care to housing and education. With help from the federal government, we worked in underprivileged areas as ombudsmen to patients and their families, and we ran health care centers to provide free services such as prenatal care.

In 1966 I went to southern California to do this sort of work. Then, in 1967 or 1968, I organized a project for the South Bronx to which we recruited students of nursing, law, dentistry, and medicine. I did that part time during medical school semesters and full time during the summers. The program heightened the sensitivity of the student participants to the problems of the urban poor, and provided real help to some of the people. To my disappointment, in those communities today circumstances appear even worse than they were then.

Among my studies, internal medicine and medical subspecialties weren't especially attractive. I appreciated their importance but there was no craft, and I liked work that required a hands-on approach. In college I had enjoyed working in construction as a framer and finish carpenter, and surgery had a similar appeal. You are more involved in the sense that your technical and creative abilities are more important to the patient's outcome than when dealing with a problem requiring purely medical management. I was not excited by all of the surgical specialties, but orthopedics was just plain appealing.

I made my decision in the third or fourth year of medical school when I was working on the orthopedic service. At Albert Einstein Medical School we had a visiting professor of orthopedics who was a very engaging person and an extraordinary teacher. I approached him after one of his lectures and asked if I could do some clinical work with him in England after he returned home. As part of my elective program, I went there for 3 months when I was a senior in medical school. It was a wonderful experience that gave me credentials, opened doors, and confirmed my career choice.

I lined up my orthopedic residency toward the end of medical school. We didn't have a match program then; it was all much less structured. Today a student must have an orthopedic program well organized by the beginning of the fourth year. The final arrangements are made midyear by means of the match program. After medical school a year of general surgery precedes the orthopedic surgery program; the two may or may not come as a package. The entire training takes 5 years. Then you may go into practice or enter a fellowship for further specialized training.

I went from medical school into a general surgical internship and residency for about a year and a half. Then I did 6 months of research before starting my clinical training in orthopedics at Harvard. Because I retained an interest in community health services issues I got to know a physician in the Department of Family and Community Medicine at the University of Massachusetts Medical Center, and while still a resident, I would go out and see patients in a clinic in downtown Worcester. That fostered my attachment to this institution, and I went from my residency to a dual appointment in the Departments of Orthopedics and of Family and Community Medicine at this center. I've been here for 16 years. When I came, the center was new and the chance to help build an institution was exciting. I picked a career in academic medicine because of the potential for achievement and influence. I felt that the rewards— professional and personal but not necessarily monetary—would be greater.

I have never contemplated a career in family and community medicine or in preventive medicine, but I have considered health care administration and policy. Although I'm not contemplating a career change just now, I haven't closed the door on other choices in the future. I remain concerned with social issues, but perhaps not as much as I should be.

I serve as an advisor to medical students. In our discussions about choosing a field, I personalize my comments by explaining why I did not want to be an internist, family practitioner, or dermatologist. Their work just did not seem to satisfy my desire for creative hands-on involvement. But I could have entered other fields such as anesthesiology or even psychiatry.

Even though it may sound as though I was on a focused pathway when I made my decision, my career could have gone in a different direction if I had found a mentor in general surgery, ophthalmology, or another area. It's an unusual student who has enough first-hand experience with a specialty and is informed enough to make the one "perfect" career choice. You look around for the best opportunities and then try to make the best decision you can. The more direct exposure you can get, the better. It is possible to make a mistake, but students should relax about it and not create a crisis. Taking the attitude that you will bloom wherever you are planted rather than searching for the ideal plot of soil probably brings greater success and comfort.

One reason for the appeal of orthopedics is that it encompasses a broad spectrum. You could be a traumatologist dealing with major life-threatening trauma on an emergency basis. You handle the problems as they come in, and you can't say that you only take care of the big toe on the right foot. This high-tension environment is demanding intellectually, emotionally, and physically, and the outcome for the patient is not always perfect. Sometimes the best care may leave significant functional deficits, whereas in another type of orthopedic practice the problems may seem easier and the functional outcome more predictable.

For example, a practice limited to arthroscopic knee surgery is very elective and relatively controlled. The patients are generally ambulatory and healthy, and although you should know about their general health status, you need not be as concerned with it because usually there are no multiple system conditions or ongoing problems. Yet each subdivision will have tense and unpredictable moments. In orthopedics you can care for adults, children, or both. You can do reconstructive work, or you can tackle more acute problems. Research has also become an increasingly important part of orthopedics. Most patient relations in orthopedics are long term. Thus, the success of a reconstructive procedure such as a hip replacement is based on the long-term outcome. Even after surgery for an acute traumatic injury both short- and long-term follow-up are necessary.

When I went into this specialty, it was looked on as less intellec-

tual than some other fields. That did not matter much to me because I was near the top of my class in college and medical school
and did not see my career choice as a symbol of accomplishment.
The orthopedists whom I came to know seemed intelligent, capable,
thoughtful, and often scholarly; the negative perception wasn't
borne out. Subsequently, orthopedics has attracted some of the best
people in medicine. It has become quite competitive, which only
breeds more excellence.

I chose orthopedics over other aspects of surgery because I liked
the craft aspect. It provides a diverse and potentially successful
armamentarium to treat sickness or injury, and there are fewer life-
threatening problems. We are not intensivists. I should mention too
that the practice of orthopedics provides a good living and, therefore,
a good quality of life. That wasn't at the top of my list, but it was a
consideration.

I do adult reconstructive surgery, mostly joint replacements. In
the time I've been at it, our techniques have changed quite a bit and
we are able to perform more difficult procedures to restore function
and relieve pain. We have become much more sophisticated about
the biomechanical aspects of the musculoskeletal system, about
rehabilitation after reconstruction, and about replacement or aug-
mentation of inadequate skeletal structure. All this is now more
exciting and challenging both intellectually and technically. However, the bureaucratic and administrative sides of medicine have
become more burdensome. I feel that we can overcome these problems by focusing more on the opportunities than on the obstacles.

I operate 2 days a week, sometimes 3. How long depends on the
nature of the case. It might be for 8 to 10 hours, and the long days
are physically wearing. On the other days, I see patients, do research, write, and tend to my administrative and educational responsibilities. I work about 65 hours a week. I used to put in more
hours, but now I take trauma call only 2–3 days a month.

I would like to have more time with my family but my professional life is extremely rewarding. I get almost enough time for my
personal needs, and during the last 3 or 4 years I have tried to spend
more time with my family. If you're not careful, medicine can con-
sume you completely. That may be good for the patients and even
good for the profession, but it leaves the other people in your life
short and increases the risk of burnout. It is important to reach a
balance.

My wife works part time as a nurse practitioner. She didn't practice at all when the children were very young. Now my daughter, 13, and my son, 10, have their own busy lives and need less parenting time. I do not think they feel that we are too involved in our work.

I would certainly recommend medicine as a career choice but with some qualifications. Some of the shine is off the jewel. My son may be interested in orthopedic sports medicine, and my daughter in architecture. I'm very glad they have goals; it's important even if they change their minds. I don't encourage them about going into medicine as much as I was encouraged because medicine is undergoing something of an industrialization and I'm not certain that it will be as attractive a career 15 years from today as it has been.

The negative changes are not cast in concrete, however. Things will get better with good leadership and sustained dedication to the service of our patients. There is room for optimism, and it is still a great privilege to be a physician. In our society entering medicine reflects a high level of accomplishment, and that should afford students great comfort and confidence. A student's anxiety over the decisions about specialties, decisions that seem so earth shaking, should be tempered by an appreciation of the great progress that he or she has already made in life. Because you are already in a good position, you are unlikely to make a very wrong decision about the rest of your career path. Regardless of whether you point your life in this professional direction or that, you are likely to be truly happy as a physician.

Chapter 18

CARDIOLOGY

This story illustrates how it is possible to be rejected from all of the medical schools to which you apply, overcome that setback, graduate as a physician, and become an expert in a rather technical clinical field. It also reflects the delicate balancing act involved in developing specialized skills while preserving one's concern for the patient as a human being.

Dr. Linda A. Pape is an associate professor of medicine in the school of medicine at the University of Massachusetts Medical Center in Worcester. A cardiologist, she devotes her professional time to teaching and patient care with a clinical emphasis on echocardiography.

Linda A. Pape, M.D., Cardiology, Academic Medical Center

One thing that I do advise students is to know yourself, be true to yourself, and don't become a person that someone else wants you to be.

Deciding to become a doctor was an "Aha!" experience for me. It started when I was out of college and working as a chemist for the Food and Drug Administration (FDA). As a child, I had no definite career plans. My parents were German immigrants with eighth-grade educations who wanted their children to go to college to better themselves. We lived on a dairy farm in upstate New York until I was 9, and then we moved to a blue collar town on Long Island, New York, where my father owned a delicatessen. The boys there gravitated toward engineering while the girls went to secretarial or nursing school or to a state teacher's college with free tuition.

I was near the top of my high school class, but I didn't know what I wanted to do and the guidance counselor was no help. Without thinking about it too much, I decided to teach elementary school. To save money, I went to Potsdam State Teachers College in upstate New York. It had a good music program and music was a major interest for me. I signed up for elementary education but the curriculum proved too superficial for my tastes, and I switched into high school science teaching. I started with a lot of chemistry because that schedule also allowed me to take music courses. By attending summer sessions I finished in 3 years. With my chemistry degree I got a job at the FDA in New York City. If I were to do it over again, I would go to a liberal arts school, take English, history, language, math, and some science, and not get pushed into career training prematurely.

At the FDA I did lab work involved in quality control. My supervisors wanted to send me to graduate school in chemistry but—and don't ask where it came from because I don't know—I finally thought, "Why don't I become a doctor?" I had always felt that the decision would just come to me sometime, and it did. Today, that's what I counsel students: the answer will come to you.

I had completed most of the course requirements for medical school but I had gone to an obscure state college and, because I hadn't worked hard enough, had ended up with a B average. So when I applied to well-known medical schools having also gotten mediocre results on the MCATs, I didn't get in anywhere—and I was shocked.

For advice, I sought out the dean at Downstate Medical School (SUNY). Mostly he probed the reason for my sudden interest in medicine, which I characterized as a late but mature decision. He was of no help so I went to see the dean at Columbia. He advised me to take a few courses at a prestigious school to show that I could make the grade, take the MCATs again, and apply to less competitive schools.

I couldn't redo my academic career, but I felt certain I could pull it back together. I took science courses at night at Columbia, got good grades, and really enjoyed the work. I like scientific inquiry but I've never been narrowly focused on science. I consider myself more a physician and a teacher than a pure scientist.

After I finished the courses at Columbia, I went to the Medical College of Pennsylvania, which at that time admitted only women and was therefore less competitive. I had never been in an all-women environment, but I felt that if that's what it took to become a doctor, so be it. As it turned out, I was happy. In 1968, when I entered medical school, medical schools had only 5–10 percent women. Things are different now, but then it was good to be in an all-women school. Now that it's 50–50, my perception is that most women students don't feel disadvantaged and are treated fairly equally; yet there is a long way to go to achieve non-sexist medical education because the teachers are left over from the older generation. Medical schools have tried to keep up with the times, but we need to see how the classes with 50 percent women will evolve.

In the past, young women were encouraged to go into teaching because it was a "nice job for a girl." You can return to it after your children are in school and you can take summers off. Now, when women go into fields other than teaching, they still seek jobs that allow them to marry and have children. When I'm asked how I did it, I say, "Don't marry someone who's not going to be a full partner. It won't work, especially in medicine." If one spouse has too demanding a schedule, the other may in effect become a single parent.

Examine your goals and balance them out. If you want children, you have to sacrifice some achievement. A few superstars manage to have five children and get elected to the National Academy of Sciences, but most of us aren't like them. People are still asking, "Why can't I be a good doctor, make a contribution, and also have a family?" That can be a tough question. No field of medicine is precluded, even surgery, but in surgery you probably have to postpone childbearing. Subspecialties within surgery allow some control over your life. (I don't know any women in cardiac surgery—that would be difficult). Some women go back to work right after delivering a child, although they may have second thoughts. After I had my second child, I took 3 months off and came back part time for a month. For me that was important, but I try to avoid imposing my views on others.

When I interviewed here for my cardiology fellowship, I was a few months pregnant and was scheduled to start my training when my daughter would be 6 months old. In talking with people in the department, I was encouraged by such statements as "I'm sorry, we have to finish up this meeting. My wife is out of town and I have to pick up my daughter from violin lessons." In that setting it was acceptable to acknowledge that you had a family whereas when I was an intern and resident, I felt that you weren't even allowed to mention it.

When I entered medical school, I was so relieved to be there that I thought I had nothing more to decide. Within a few months, I realized that I had more decisions to make. I gravitated toward the "liberal arts" choice, internal medicine—the direction for people who don't want to make a decision just yet and who are interested in many different things. For some fields, like eye surgery, you had to decide years in advance. I didn't know that I did not want to be an eye surgeon, but there wasn't much exposure to those subspecialties, so I stayed with the broad-based possibilities.

During the third-year clerkships my interest crystallized almost by elimination. My idea of being a doctor was best embodied by internal medicine. Family medicine didn't exist yet, so the general choices came down to internal medicine, surgery, and pediatrics— and I wasn't very excited by pediatrics or surgery. It had to do with the strong people on the faculty with whom I could identify and the intellectual content of the daily discourse. In my fourth year, I took primarily medicine electives plus a 9-week surgical clerkship at the Brigham in Boston. In cardiology I had some wonderful teachers who planted the seeds of my interest in that area. I liked the way they thought, the detective work of putting things together, the approach to examining the patient, and the physiology. They were clinically oriented and were just starting to do echocardiograms.

I stayed at the Medical College of Pennsylvania for my 3 years of residency training in general internal medicine. Although I continued to have an interest in cardiology, I didn't have specific plans to become a cardiologist. My husband, whom I had married during my fourth year of medical school, and I decided together to stay in Philadelphia to give us both more options.

The next decision after residency training involved a fellowship. My husband was finishing his graduate work in German literature. He had originally planned to do his graduate work at Yale, but my career choice had steered him back to Princeton and so now it was his turn to decide where we would land. I did not apply for a fellowship right away and we ended up in Middlebury, Vermont, where he taught and I got pregnant. I couldn't find any work in medicine—the medical school was too far away. In retrospect, taking a year out wasn't so terrible. In the long run, it doesn't make any difference. But you shouldn't take a year off before your internship; you should get that over with.

When I applied for a fellowship, I chose cardiology. I became aware that UMass in Worcester was opening a new hospital and I had heard of its new head of cardiology when he had been at the Brigham during my fourth-year clerkship there, so I came down to see the place. The hospital wasn't even open but the program was starting. I met the group and was offered their fellowship. I had two options: sign on for a promising though not yet established new program, or wait a year to get back into the regular application cycle. Hoping for the best, I signed up at UMass for the next July.

By the time I settled on a fellowship it was clear to me that I wanted to stay in an academic setting and enjoy teaching, patient care, research, and continued learning. I now have a small, long-term practice, and I have patients whom I see on a limited basis as they stay affiliated with their primary doctors. They know my children from pictures; and when I was seriously ill, they wrote frequent letters. I get enough of that sort of long-term continuity to derive great pleasure from it. I also see many new patients briefly. For them I do the testing, try to figure out the diagnosis, refer them to surgery, and then maybe follow them periodically at a distance through their internist or family doctor. I try not to become their primary physician.

When I started the 2-year cardiology fellowship, I didn't feel pressure to find a niche right away. I didn't want to be procedure-oriented. Because I liked diagnostic puzzles and challenges, I enjoyed the catheterization lab since it gives you the chance to question and examine a patient and find out the answer. I liked it, but I didn't want to do it year in and year out. Today, we have six full-time cath people here. They receive many prescreened patients and many undiagnosed patients. As they become more subspecialized for doing balloon angioplasties and the like, doctors send them patients for angioplasty who have been worked up extensively.

With all of this specialization, there's a risk of fragmentation of the patient. As people become good at what they do, they are the ones you want to perform the highly technical procedures. But patients still need the clinical cardiologist to act as their advocate, help them through the maze, see them in the clinic first, decide on a course of investigation, distill the results of the consultation, refer them to the cath lab, and interpret those results.

I ended up specializing in echocardiography, a fairly technical diagnostic tool. Echo was a regular rotation during my fellowship. I didn't take additional training; I just put in extra time. At first, I tried to keep my options open. I spent my third year in the dog lab and also toyed with the idea of cardiopathology. Echo offered me the chance to get into a diagnostic area that solves clinical problems and is a good tool for looking at the physiology of the circulation. The opportunity to stay on arose and, because of my interest and the expanding possibilities in the division, I joined the faculty. I finished my fellowship in 1979, and I've been in practice since then. Today I still see general cardiology patients referred for diagnostic evaluation and I do echo training for the fellows. My area of diagnostic work is echocardiography, and I participate in the general teaching consultative service. I also teach physical diagnosis and gross anatomy of the heart. My research relates to the use of echocardiography as a tool for studying left ventricular hypertrophy and myocardial infarction.

To explore something a little more basic, I'm about to take my first sabbatical. My husband, who teaches college German and is taking a leave of absence, our 15-year-old daughter, our 7-year-old son, and I are going to Freiburg, Germany. There I will work on the relation between the coronary endothelium and arteriosclerosis, a hot topic. I will also participate in research protocols involving intravascular ultrasound.

I want to see if the new area is interesting and whether I might want to continue working in it after I return. I don't enjoy administrative duties enough to go in that direction. I have the feeling that sometime in the next 5 or 10 years I'd like to try to make a broader impact on the way medicine works, maybe with respect to the position of women in society or other social issues; it hasn't gelled yet. I may do something of that nature along with what I'm doing now.

At this point, both of my children are definite about not going into medicine. I think it's because they don't want to go through what they have seen me experience. Even now, when my work load is lighter, I take calls on weekends and nights. So I stay neutral about their future plans. I have no emotional investment in their becoming doctors, but if they wanted to do it, it would be a wonderful career.

As I care for my patients, I appreciate the good we do in ministering to the sick and in interacting with them. I would like all doctors to be sufficiently available to their patients, but part of me doesn't want to give over my entire life to it. In medicine there are deep tensions between professional and personal life. Some doctors appear to want little contact with patients in order to pursue a regular home life or research interests; but if too many of them feel this way who will take care of sick people?

Look within the academic community. To whom can we refer our patients? To whom do we want to go ourselves? Even here at our institution the number of "real doctors" is diminishing as we become more research-oriented. Off campus, there still are "real" doctors who are available to their patients, but their practices are changing too. They may not always be covering when a patient calls. I admire the commitment of some family practitioners I know, but that commitment can be overwhelming and can preclude a normal family life. The doctor who is the wonderful available doctor is probably not that to his or her family. It's a dilemma.

Discussions such as these should be helpful to many students as they go about choosing their career directions. The way people arrive at their decisions has always interested me because my approach has been one of almost stumbling into them. My advice is to be careful not to push people too early. Don't push little kids into reading, don't push high school students into picking a job, and don't push medical students into choosing a career path too soon. There should be enough time for people to evolve and find a niche—or even not find one. I encourage students to realize that their lives do not rest on a single decision like picking a residency. There are always other choices and other options. If you have the potential and if you have reasonably good luck, those things will come to you.

There's too little time for growth as a person outside of medicine because you can't do everything. My husband and I have probably advanced less quickly in our professions than we might have if we had not had children. There are other things we'd like to be doing. We talk about taking music lessons. He keeps me aware of new books to read, and I make some time to read them. But many things that I'd like to do I never will.

When my son was 8 months old, I was diagnosed as having diffuse histiocytic lymphoma. I underwent surgery and then chemotherapy. I had a 50–50 likelihood of surviving, and from the early news I got I thought I was probably going to die. It's now years later and I'm doing fine, with no evidence of disease. I try not to talk about my medical experience too much because I don't want to make people feel uncomfortable. Yet I can relate to things in a different way.

When I was in chemotherapy, I wished I could use the experience to help my patients. Some of them who knew I was ill and out of practice for a year showed, through writing letters and other acts, how much they cared about me. My situation gave them permission to be sympathetic to their doctor. Sometimes I relate my experience to them to help them a bit. In that way, it's been useful. That's about as far as I've gone with it with patients.

I also tried to figure out how to convey to medical students the experience of being a doctor who becomes a patient and goes through major difficulties. It could be helpful to them, but I haven't discovered how to make it useful. Being a patient is a valuable experience. Some students aren't very sympathetic people, and maybe my story wouldn't help them at all. But if you're an empathetic person, it helps a lot.

Like everyone, I would just as soon have done without the whole ordeal. There were times when I would say to my husband, "Damn it, if I die next week and I didn't do this or that, I am going to be really angry, so I better make time for it." I would remind myself about that again and again. The first few years you feel fragile and worry that you're never going to get a chance to do those things. Then you start to feel your old cocky self. That's the good news. You feel normal again. But you do keep the one-day-at-a-time feeling, not that it hangs like a cloud over you. It's a little reminder to enjoy life.

One thing that I do advise students is to know yourself, be true to yourself, and don't become a person that someone else wants you to be. The other thing I try to do is to talk with them about their own individual concerns. Students come to me with such problems as how to make a good transition into medicine—a world they see as alien. For students who have had no prior contact with medicine, we show them that we value those attributes that lay people used to ascribe to physicians. By caring for medical students, we demonstrate that caring for one another is important. It sounds trite, but it is essential to ensure that the students passing through our lives are not so beaten by the time they leave training that they can't care about patients anymore.

I can take a lot of time with my patients because I'm not in a place that's scheduling a patient for me every 10 minutes, which does happen with doctors in HMOs. We need a system that allows people adequate compensation but doesn't overcompensate for the wrong things. I do not want to encourage a clock-punching mentality in which the doctors don't care one way or the other and no longer feel any excitement about their work. You do not want to take the joy out of medicine or some of the incentives for all of the hard work either. Despite the problems, I'm happy to be a doctor.

Chapter 19

CLINICAL RESEARCH

Some physicians go to medical school intending to immerse themselves in patient care and later gravitate into a research career in response to unexpected external factors. Others sense from their early youth that an inner need to engage in a quest for new knowledge, either at the laboratory bench or at the bedside, is a compelling element of their emotional makeup. Regardless of when it is made, the decision to follow a research career requires a heavy dose of self-confidence because the gratification of successful achievement may not come until long after the career path has been chosen and other opportunities have been foregone. Dr. Sullivan says, "Although part of my interest in medicine came out of wanting to help the sick, part of it was also the science, the idea of discovery." But his entry into the research world was not smooth or easy in its initial phases.

Dr. John L. Sullivan is a professor of pediatrics and director of the Division of Rheumatology and Immunology at the medical school of the University of Massachusetts Medical Center in Worcester.

**John L. Sullivan, M.D., Pediatric Immunology,
Clinical Research, Academic Medical Center**

I just want to make some solid and important contributions and have my legacy be that John Sullivan was a pediatrician

*and a viral immunologist who helped us to understand this
and that. I also want to help the kids with the diseases I've
tackled.*

I was born and raised in Plattsburg, New York. My great uncle
was a country doctor in Norfolk, New York, near the Canadian
border. When he moved there, the people were suffering from cal-
cium deficiency, so he started a dairy farm to provide milk. Because
of stories about my uncle's practice and because of my interest in
science, I decided in high school to pursue a premedical program in
college. I was the first one in my family to go to college.

During summers in high school, I was a farm worker, a short-
order cook, a waiter, and a railroad construction worker. In my
junior year of college I got a job for a year and a half in the hospital
labs at the nearby Upstate (SUNY–Syracuse) Medical School. They
trained about 12 of us to do the stat lab work nights and weekends.
That fantastic experience cemented my feelings about medicine.
The emergency room residents taught us how to suture and let us
do an occasional simple scalp laceration. Boy, did that get the juices
flowing!

Although part of my interest in medicine came from wanting to
help the sick, part of it was also the science, the idea of discovery.
In college, I did extra work with an organic chemist who was synthe-
sizing new compounds for possible use against cancer. I was excited
by thinking about and helping to create something of potential benefit to patients with cancer.

I majored in biology and had good exam scores, but I didn't do
well on my MCATs. I wanted to go to Upstate because as a state
school it had low tuition. I was interviewed by almost every medical
school to which I applied and felt confident about being accepted
somewhere. But warning signals came my way. In one interview an
elderly man told me that my grades and scores led him to believe
that I was an overachiever and unlikely to make it through medical
school. I spent much of my senior year waiting for letters from
medical schools, but I wasn't accepted by a single one. It was terrible! By May I had wound up on a couple of waiting lists and had to
face the decision of what to do. I still wanted to go to medical school
but decided to pursue a PhD first.

I was admitted into the biochemistry PhD program but I needed
to make up courses in advanced calculus and physical chemistry. I

started in the Syracuse University summer session, but the physical chemistry course was too difficult on an accelerated schedule. I dropped it but did well in the advanced calculus course. I got married that summer to Lynn, who is from Lemoyne, the college I'd attended. I was still working in the hospital lab at night and found a second job selling shoes. In late August, a student failed to show up for the medical school's orientation day; I learned from a call to me at the shoe store that I was admitted to medical school. I started out feeling like the last one accepted, the least bright member of the class. All through the first semester I was concerned about flunking out. Five schools had told me I couldn't hack it and I had a lot to prove to myself. It was difficult, but it worked out well.

In freshman year, we were assigned to faculty advisors through a lottery. As student 104 our of 105, my choice was between a radiologist and a pediatrician. I picked the pediatrician, and he helped to determine my future course in medicine. A general pediatrician who'd had on-the-job training in hematology, he participated in a high school program for unwed pregnant students. Between my first and second years, I worked with him doing physical exams and developmental assessments of the students' babies.

During the summer between second and third year, I did another pediatric fellowship in hematology with my advisor and his colleague — an authentic hematologist — in which I cared for kids with leukemia and other hematologic disorders. I met many pediatricians and in my third-year rotations, despite enjoying medicine, I decided that pediatrics was for me. The fourth year was all electives, and the program I designed turned out to be the equivalent of a pediatric internship. Some people do the opposite and take electives outside their chosen field, but that seemed silly. After all, you're never going to use the other stuff again so why not go ahead and learn what you are going to use in your own field?

In the beginning of my senior year, a pediatric infectious disease specialist directed me into a project evaluating a new treatment for impetigo. Infectious disease interested me and after sampling other fields I decided to proceed with pediatrics, obtain experience in infectious disease, and do research in an academic setting. I liked the people in the subspecialties, who in pediatrics are mostly university-based. Because Dr. Paul Parkman, the discoverer of the rubella virus, was an alumnus of Upstate Medical Center and assistant director of the Bureau of Biologics at the NIH, I was encouraged to try for a research assignment at the NIH to get the experience needed for academic medicine.

I applied for a matching program at NIH that permitted you to complete a 3-year residency and then go to work in an NIH research lab. I interviewed for a slot in a virus lab. You got the results as you were about to start your internship. For my internship I chose the University of Washington because I thought I should get another view of the world. While we were driving west to start my internship, I learned from a phone call back to Syracuse that I had matched but that I would have to start after only 1 year of clinical training. The position was in a virology research lab in the Bureau of Biologics on NIH's main campus. I accepted with my car motor running.

Going to Seattle knowing that I was headed for a virus research lab at the end of the year provided a carrot at the end of the stick. After being constantly awakened at 3 in the morning to see runny-nosed kids in the emergency room, I was ready for a break. In effect, it was my second year of internship because of my experience in the fourth year of medical school.

A fellow intern from the University of Alabama had taken time off from medical school to go to Australia to pursue a masters degree in immunology. We sometimes chatted in the library. I talked about infectious disease and he talked about immunology. He raised my interest because in 1972 immunology was just blossoming. As a result, when I went to the NIH I decided to study how viruses interact with the immune system, a subject about which not much was known.

I went into a traditional lab with people doing primarily vaccine-oriented virology; they didn't have a strong background in immunology. However, on the NIH campus there was a vast informal immunology program in the night courses and in the noontime journal clubs. One course covered basic immunology, another immunogenetics, another immunodeficiencies, and so on. I took every course I could and started thinking about unanswered questions.

I began working on a measles virus, trying to find out what cells it infected in the immune system and what effects it had on immune reactivity. The people in my lab helped me grow the virus, but they didn't know much about T cells and B cells. I learned that from my mentors, the world leaders who taught in the night courses. When you needed help, you could always turn to them.

I went into the lab totally unprepared for full-time bench research. I had grown up in the clinical environment where you get daily gratification from making diagnoses and interacting with patients. Having no knowledge of virology and immunology, I worked 7 days a week. After a year I had nothing to show for it; no one even told me I was doing a good job. I had no papers to submit for publication and no data to present at a national meeting. No one told me not to expect much more from 1 year.

Toward year's end, I decided that I had been unsuccessful because I was in a lousy lab with second-rate people and I wasn't going to waste any more time. I left the lab, went home for a few days, and then called my infectious disease mentor in Syracuse and said, "These people here are lousy and I want out." I was even willing to transfer and spend my remaining 2 years of obligated service in the National Health Service Corps taking care of the poor and disadvantaged. Then my mentor said, "John, grow up, will you?" I hated him at that moment but I decided to stay put.

I moped around for another day or two and returned to the lab. What followed was unbelievable. Out of the next 2 years came 10 good papers. It was hard to leave when my time was up. We were the first to show that the measles virus is T cell–trophic, that it prefers to replicate in T cells, and that monocytes of newborn humans are more permissive for viral replication than monocytes from adults. The work garnered the attention of leaders in the field. I was shocked that I'd come so close to quitting. I had learned that when physicians come into a laboratory from their clinical training, it is essential to prepare them properly for the experience and to warn them not to become discouraged if their hard work produces only meager results.

Measles was only part of this blossoming field. I also worked on the influenza and Epstein–Barr (E–B) viruses. Our E–B virus paper was one of the seminal papers on cell-mediated cellular toxicity and was published in the *New England Journal of Medicine*. It was as though everything we touched turned to gold.

Another lesson I learned was that when a physician comes into the lab, you must give that person a problem that will work out, even if it isn't earth shattering. In my case, I picked my own projects, and their successful outcome was pure luck. Although I didn't have formal research training, there were enough opportunities to acquire the skills. That period at NIH was the heyday of the "two-year man," people like myself. Perhaps because of the Vietnam War, the NIH matching program was overfilled with embryonic physician–scientists. Now they have so few applicants they're thinking of eliminating the program.

It's a major problem that I just don't understand. I can't accept the argument that students come out of medical school so heavily in debt that they can't afford to take 2 years off; most state medical schools have reasonable tuition. I don't know who will teach medicine in the future. Our clinical faculty will simply be members of group practice clinics. They will be well-trained clinical subspecialists, but they won't be able to think and teach like physician–investigators.

After I left the NIH, I returned to the University of Washington, did one more year of clinical residency, and then stayed for a 2-year NIH research fellowship in pediatric immunology and rheumatology. I returned to a project from my Bethesda days by using E–B virus to create B-cell lines from the hospital's large population of patients with immunodeficiencies to try to figure out what the immunologic defect was in those patients.

I did other related projects and came to realize that I liked thinking about clinical immunodeficiencies. So I decided to be a pediatric immunologist who concentrated on viral interactions with the immune system. I have attacked problems at a fundamental level but I have not become a molecular biologist; I am a clinical investigator. I can't compete with the molecular biologists who never go to clinic, even the MDs among them. They can devote all their time and energy to precisely defined and limited areas. I prefer working with people and trying to learn about the mechanisms that cause human disease. Molecular types think in terms of biochemical signals inside a cell and how a message gets from one molecule to another. I want to know what happens in the whole organism, and that's where they can't compete with me.

For instance, they might not have gotten involved with the kid I saw here with generalized chicken pox. She would have died if we hadn't admitted her to the ICU, put her on a respirator, and treated her with an antiviral drug that works against herpes viruses. When she was over the acute illness, I went after the reason why she had almost died of chicken pox. We started to explore the different components of her immune system and finally found that she had a complete absence of natural killer (NK) cells.

She is the first patient ever described with this complete deficiency, which fits beautifully with all the studies done on the consequences of viral infections in mice with NK cell defects. My patient went on to contract a series of life-threatening disseminated viral infections. We learned that because she doesn't have NK cells, she can't control viral replication in the early phases of an infection and is overwhelmed by the virus. However, if we can keep her alive in the first week or two, her B cells and T cells will kick in, and then she will make a normal immune response and recover. The role of NK cells had been shown in mice; we found that the same was true for humans.

So far, the only preventive thing we can do for her is to give monthly infusions of high doses of gamma globulin to try to protect her against other viral infections. Together with a colleague at Memorial Sloan-Kettering, we have considered a marrow transplant. She has a sibling with an HLA-matched marrow, but even under such circumstances, there have been severe reactions and we're waiting. As she waits, we're learning more and more about NK cells. This is the kind of clinical investigation I do.

I didn't stay in Seattle after I finished my fellowship because they did not have an abundance of resources for young people. I ended up with three job offers: Michigan, Ohio, and Massachusetts. At the UMass medical school in Worcester the pediatrics chairman had received his MD from Syracuse, knew my mentors there, and was interested in talking to me. He scheduled me for a talk at an affiliated hospital and reserved a room at a budget motel. My plane was late and I reached the motel at midnight. It was closed up tight and when the manager finally appeared and unchained the six locks on her door, she told me that my reservation had not been guaranteed and the last room had been given away. I finally found another place and got to bed at 3 o'clock in the morning. Early next day, my host came by and took me to the hospital. We went to a dingy little conference room where I gave my talk to three residents who were half asleep. Then we went to the brand new buildings of the medical school and its hospital, and despite mud all around the place, you could walk down halls and halls of empty new labs.

By contrast, in Ohio, they did their homework and wined and dined me. At the children's hospital they showed me an adjoining empty four-floor research building. The dean, who ran the rhinovirus reference laboratory for the World Health Organization, offered me "whatever space" I wanted and said he would make me chief of allergy, immunology, and rheumatology. I gave grand rounds and enjoyed a top-notch academic reception.

But when I looked around I discovered that everybody was taking care of patients and nobody was doing investigative work. I felt that I would get swallowed up as the one person who wanted to get a lab going. I finally reasoned that because there weren't any patients at UMass yet, and because their labs were empty, I could come in and get my research going before the pull of the clinical work encroached on my lab time. Besides, it was close to my family.

I was confident that I could get started on my own. A fellow in the UMass pathology department had reported three families in which boys had become infected with the E–B virus and had died or become immunodeficient. It's called the X-linked lymphoproliferative syndrome. The fellow was a guru in pathology but had no background in immunology, so we teamed up. It was a perfect way to kick off my interest in viruses and the immune system.

We started doing lots of E–B virus work, and I set up a clinic at the UMass campus in Amherst. A nurse practitioner there sees students with mononucleosis, and that's where we get our clinical material. We're trying to work out the details of the cellular immune response in that infection. The E–B virus is a real pathogen in immunodeficient patients. For example, patients whose immune systems are depressed in preparation for bone marrow and liver transplants are susceptible to E–B virus-induced lymphoproliferative disorders. Most people who have mono get over it and that's that. We wanted to identify what in the immune response is important for recovering from the infection and what defects occur in immunodeficient patients.

In research you need a theme, and mine is viruses interacting with the immune system. The two viruses on which I now have a portfolio are E–B and HIV. E–B produces an acute viral infection that ends up in lifelong latency and can create exacerbations for certain people. HIV produces an acute infection that ends up as a persistent active viral infection. We contrast and compare what happens in E–B and HIV. I could envision spending the rest of my research career this way, but working in the trenches is becoming a battle. Keeping a research operation funded is difficult, even in the best of hands. We are currently well funded and recently I decided to give it 5 more years. I'll be 50 then and might start thinking about something else.

I don't know what, though. Originally, my long-term plan was to become a department chairman, but I'm less enamored with that now because the resources are thin. In my clinical research I have interacted with biotechnology and pharmaceutical companies, and I might try something in their world. Depending on what happens in 5 years, becoming scientific dean of an institution is another possibility. I like inspiring people to work together. I'm not sure I could walk away from lab work, but I begin to think it's quite possible when I'm rewriting a grant application, or writing a new application because when my two grants get renewed they're cut so drastically that they won't pay for the work to be done.

It's a question of how long a person can continue to devote 60–70 hours a week to a career. That expenditure of energy burns people out. I am still 100 percent enthusiastic when I talk to my trainees, though. I think a career in science is fantastic. Yet the difficulties of getting support to run a decent lab will probably make the next couple of years a trying time in biomedical research. Eventually it should turn around because the problem is appreciated. It will never be like the heyday of the 1960s, but it may become easier to maintain productive research programs. If that happens, I'll stay with it.

At a recent social function I met an internist who said he's looking for something else to do because he's so fed up with medicine that he's even pleased his kids are not going into it. I told him I had a hard time believing he meant what he was saying. I love medicine and would be delighted if my daughter, who is considering a medical career, decided to pursue it. That doctor had been in practice for 26 years. I can understand his burning out and wanting to do something else, but for him to look back on his career and see nothing worthwhile in it is tragic. I still think it is the highest profession.

If my daughter wanted to go into clinical research, I would tell her that when you're young and full of vim and vigor, you can do it. The question is how long you can keep up the pace. Some people can keep going indefinitely; look at my colleague down the hall who must be near 70. He has a competitive research grant at a time when it's very difficult, when study sections are looking critically at each award. He continues to love his work and is enthusiastic about what he does. It's easier to do that with a small operation like his. Ours has grown so big it has a million dollar annual personnel budget. One solution is to shrink our lab, and I may do that.

New scientific contributions will come from the young people who are now in training. Many young people in our lab are growing and developing and will carry on our line of investigation. We must see to it that they get the tools they need. The concern today is whether we will continue to have enough young people to train. I hope so, but when NIH talks about closing their matching program because they don't have applications, that's worrisome.

Clinical investigators must limit their patient time, and I do no more than half a day a week. I carry patients on a long-term basis because the diseases I'm studying are chronic. The four of us in my division are all investigators, we all work in the clinic, and we cover for each other. We also have two nurse practitioners who are the first line of defense. I don't do any more hands-on lab work. We have a formal lab meeting every Monday, and I devote Friday afternoons to individual project meetings. I walk through the lab a lot and talk with people about their experiments. Everyone presents his or her work regularly so that everybody knows what everybody else is doing and no one works in isolation. I spend a lot of time on grant proposals, administrative work, and off-campus travel.

We helped to design a new drug for treating AIDS and we've taken it into the clinic for evaluation. To do this, we have satellite clinics around the state as part of an NIH-funded network, and I go to those clinics. I also serve on an NIH study section three times a year. I go to meetings about AIDS clinical trials three times a year, as well as to other clinical meetings and research meetings to exchange information and ideas. I'm away about 1 day a week, but I spend most of my time in research. I am board-certified as a pediatric allergist and immunologist, but I do not cover attending rounds in general pediatrics any more. One of the things on my list for the future is to spend some time with the medical school admissions committee.

As for personal life, I'm big on sports, as a participant and as a spectator. I like to read, in a hodge-podge way. My wonderful wife is a specialist in early education and has been in the local Head Start program for many years. I have two daughters, the youngest of whom is a junior in high school. However, my family has paid a price for my career choice. While I've tried to balance things, I've put my profession first. So far, things have worked out pretty well and, fortunately, everyone has held together.

I don't see how medicine can be a 40-hour-a-week job, regardless of which aspect you choose. If people go into medicine looking for a rewarding lifestyle, they must realize that physicians are indeed rewarded well financially, despite the moaning and groaning, and one can't expect that kind of reward without giving more of oneself than in most other professions.

As for what's driven me, I've never had pretenses about a Nobel Prize or anything like that. I just want to make some solid and important contributions and have my legacy be that John Sullivan was a pediatrician and a viral immunologist who helped us to understand this and that. I also want to help the kids with the diseases I've tackled. Before I quit, I want to figure out the X-linked lymphoproliferative syndrome and fix it. Right now, it's at the molecular genetics level and a collaborator in Boston is close to having the gene. When he does, we'll go after the product that the gene makes and its role in the workings of the immune system. Then we'll come up with the right treatment. That pretty much covers the next 5 years.

The key point is to enjoy what you choose. If my first adviser, the pediatrician, had been an SOB or if we had gotten along poorly, I probably would have turned to something else. But I enjoyed the experience with him, and that was the key. Medicine today is exciting to me. I love what I do and can't think of any path that I might have taken instead. There is no magic recipe for success.

Part Three

WHICH PERSON FOR WHICH PATH? REFLECTIONS OF TRAINING PROGRAM DIRECTORS

The director of a residency training program takes on various responsibilities. There is the primary responsibility to society to turn out physicians who are competent practitioners of their disciplines. There is an unwritten contract with society that the training program will do its best not to produce a physician who is warped or impaired by a deep-rooted personality defect or by an addiction to alcohol or narcotics, and who therefore constitutes a threat to his or her patients. There is a major responsibility to the resident trainees to provide them with the best possible opportunities to develop their existing talents, to acquire new skills, to learn to make wise and prudent clinical decisions, to mature as human beings, and to find an appropriate place in the world of medicine. There is a responsibility to the hospital in which the training program is conducted to provide the institution with residents who can perform their clinical duties well, who will adapt congenially to the social sphere of the hospital, and who will not disrupt the work of the staff. More than ever these days, there is yet another responsibility, a duty to the economics of the country to avoid wasteful or questionably productive expenditures. There is a duty to the art of medicine to preserve its values and culture by transmitting them to the next generation of practitioners through the residents in the program. Finally, there is a responsibility to the intellectual content of medicine to prepare residents to adapt intelligently to new ideas, new methodologies, and new insights, so that medicine does not become fossilized within the boundaries of today's knowledge.

This is no easy task and the role of residency director can be challenging. I thought it would be interesting to talk with several physicians who have taken on the assignment and to explore with them their criteria for selecting residents. As well, I wanted to know about their experiences with residents who found that they had entered a field that wasn't quite right for them. Finally, I thought it would be helpful to learn something about the people who become directors of residency programs, and so their own stories have been added to the group.

Chapter 20

MEDICINE

Dr. David Clive is a nephrologist at the school of medicine of the University of Massachusetts Medical Center in Worcester. He is an associate professor of medicine and has been the director of the residency program in internal medicine for almost a decade. He devotes his time to clinical care and teaching.

David Clive, M.D., Nephrologist, Academic Medical Center

You have to reflect deeply on what you regarded as the positive experiences in your medical school life and on why they felt positive. For example, if the best experience was delivering a baby, that may tell you something. But if your most meaningful experience was spending time at the bedside of someone dying of colon cancer, that tells you something else. We must listen to such experiential signals.

As the director of the internal medicine residency program, my responsibility is to oversee the educational experiences of our trainees during the 1 to 3 years they spend with us. They fall into two groups: first are the people who are spending 1 year in a "preliminary" internal medicine internship before departing for other areas of training such as ophthalmology, neurology, radiology, dermatology, anesthesiology, and so forth (I think that underscores how basic internal medicine is to other medical fields); the second group is the "categorical trainees," people who intend to become board-certified in internal medicine. After they have spent 3 years with us, they either go into the practice of general internal medicine, which might be called primary care internal medicine, or seek further training in a subspecialty of medicine. My job is to make sure that the variety of experiences that they have in our program will meet their needs as future internists.

I also help to select and recruit residents who during their preliminary year with us have already lined up their specialized program. That program is selected in the match at the same time as their medicine position or earlier. Nowadays preliminary internships in internal medicine are readily available; to my knowledge, most accredited programs will suffice. Most people who get into the highly sought radiology or dermatology residencies are competitive for a good internal medicine preliminary internship. In fact I have seen individuals get accepted into a preliminary medicine program and fail to match in a specialty program. More often, they have elected to stay on with us and get their boards in internal medicine. If they do a good job in a preliminary internship, we will do whatever we can to retain them in our program. It's much tighter in surgery because surgical programs are more apt to narrow down the number of trainees as the years go by.

By and large, a medical student must reach a decision about trying for fields such as ophthalmology, radiology, dermatology, and neurology sometime between the third and the beginning of the fourth year. You ought to get to know the corresponding specialists at your parent institution because you will need strong recommendations from them. As an example, dermatology is quite competitive, and someone interested in it would do well to meet the main academic dermatologists at their parent medical school—not just for letters of recommendation, but for experience in which they can excel and show prospective section heads elsewhere what they can do. This can be done in the third year or early in the fourth. The problem is, I have no idea how someone can know in the beginning of the third year of medical school that he or she definitely wants to become a dermatologist or an ophthalmologist.

Having reviewed almost 1,000 personal statements of internship applicants during the past couple of years, I can tell you that only a few have had personal experiences early in medical school or earlier in life that have determined their choice. For example, I know a physician whose mother died of lupus when he was a small boy. After that his mission in life was to become a rheumatologist.

Sometimes an early choice is inspired by a role model, someone who impresses you tremendously and whom you want to emulate. That can happen before medical school if there is a physician in the family because families provide strong role models. I've met people who remember with great affection their childhood doctor, or the doctor who set their fracture when they were on the football team. Certainly you can meet powerful role models early in medical school.

People may have a strong response to a discipline itself. Many prospective interns have told me that in medical school it was the gastroenterology or the infectious disease lectures that they found most interesting. Some people have a differential response to one field in contrast to another, which can happen quite early, although it didn't in my case.

Other factors, such as political or even religious considerations, can come into play. These days I see people who are interested in AIDS mainly because of the enormity of the problem. Almost as a matter of social conscience, they want to go into infectious diseases and be a part of the solution to this gigantic problem. There are many individuals with a missionary's view of medicine, people who intend to practice in the inner city or in a third-world country.

Feelings of this sort can lead to many possibilities. Family practice is a definite alternative for people like that because it produces trainees prepared to provide most medical services for a group of clinically underserved people. Others may be well advised to pursue special training programs in tropical and geographic medicine. You can probably enter these fields after a standard medical residency, which enables you to make the choice after obtaining a good grounding in general internal medicine.

Then there are the people whose motivations are difficult to figure out. What impelled them to gravitate to neurology, dermatology, or what have you? Some people are better suited for one area than another, making the choice of a training program intimidating to someone who is worried about going into the wrong field. That's okay; people can and do make changes. Not only are decisions not irrevocable, but the 1 or 2 years of training in an area you subsequently decide to leave will benefit you in some way. I've known about a dozen people who have come to internal medicine training and then decided to do something totally different. One went into anesthesiology and several were late converts to dermatology. I think lifestyle may have had something to do with it. Without wanting to make value judgments about how noble the different specialties are, I think internal medicine involves more personal sacrifice than many other fields.

Another field that has opened up and gained legitimacy is emergency medicine. Although there is a high degree of acuity and intensity to the work, it is scheduled shift work, which makes it appealing to a lot of people. In emergency medicine, however, you sacrifice "longitudinality" of patient care, which some people regard as the most rewarding aspect of medicine. In internal medicine, as opposed to emergency medicine and most surgical specialties, you are more likely to get to see your patients over years as they go through problems and changes, and to minister to them, perhaps for a chronic illness, with prolonged contact.

In my subspecialty, nephrology, many patients have a chronic problem that I can treat and manage but cannot cure. Among the positive aspects of this is getting to know my patient and his or her family. You are an important person to them and are always there for them. It's a difficult challenge. In many instances, doing technical procedures probably doesn't require a medical degree, but to understand another person's emotional and physical needs, and to be competent to optimize and individualize the medical care, is what separates physicians from technicians.

Some people feel negative about internal medicine because they see it as caring primarily for an aging population for whom you can do little. Caring for the aging is a lot like caring for the chronically ill. It's harder and much more challenging to care for people you can't cure than it is to care for people who can be cured in a quick interaction of some kind, but it's rewarding to do something difficult well. At times it gets me down and I may even lose sight of the rewards, but then I remind myself that what I'm doing is meaningful and compassionate.

To dissect out the factors that differentiate whether you belong in longitudinal care or episodic care is not easy. It requires knowing what kind of rewards make you feel good in life. Someone who prefers immediate, tangible gratification may not do well in internal medicine or psychiatry, for example. Someone who values rewards from within probably belongs in internal medicine. It requires maturity and self-insight to know where you fit in.

You have to reflect deeply on what you regarded as the positive experiences in your medical school life and on why they felt positive. For example, if the best experience was delivering a baby, that may tell you something. But if your most meaningful experience was spending time at the bedside of someone dying of colon cancer, that tells you something else. We must listen to such experiential signals.

You may be able to gain insight by looking back on your life, on your interests and hobbies. If you are a cerebral person who likes to read and ponder, that might incline you toward a more cognitive-oriented field like internal medicine, whereas if you are a doer, in the sense of being an athlete, or someone whose hobby is making things, as in carpentry and woodworking, that may push you to a more technical specialty. These are obvious signals, but they can have merit.

Students can sculpt their own curriculum somewhat more than they may realize. Medical students sometimes ask me if they can attend my clinic for an afternoon even if they are not on an assigned rotation with me, and I welcome them. They're trying to expose themselves to an experience that may help them arrive at a career decision. By and large, faculty are glad to help. There's much to be learned from observing people already working in a field and getting an inkling of what it's like to be them.

As for encountering residents in our training program who appear to have made a wrong decision, that is uncommon in internal medicine. It is so broad a field that there's something in it for almost everyone. I can remember only one person who decided to drop out of our program early on, and it was a wise decision. This person, who would have been unhappy in almost any area of clinical medicine, went into pathology, a field more removed from patient care. His approach to clinical problems was so ruminative that he belonged in a lab, peering through a microscope, getting up, consulting a book, coming back, thinking about the problem, and making a decision in a more cerebral and abstract sense. He also seemed to find clinical interaction and minute-to-minute decisions extremely taxing. The realization should have come earlier than it did because he dropped out within a month or two of starting the residency program, which is unusual and surprised us so much that we called his medical school dean and talked to his mentors, which is when retrospectively we gained a better notion of his true personality.

In evaluating candidates for our program, we look for bright people. You can get a sense of how bright people are from their paper credentials—the letters of recommendation and the transcripts. What is hard to glean from paper credentials is what people are like in regard to what are often called the "humanistic qualities." I'm not crazy about the term, but it is intended to cover such intangible qualities as maturity, compassion, depth, capacity to work well with others, and even articulateness.

Anyone can jerk around the paper credentials system. It's easy for an applicant to get help with writing one of those eloquent little biographic statements. In soliciting letters of recommendation you select only people who will go to bat for you. Our only shot at sizing up maturity and sincerity is during the interview, and that's daunting because we have no more than 30 minutes. But other people meet the candidates during a day's visit, and their informal interactions are helpful to us—the secretary in the residency office and the other residents who show candidates around the medical center. We have plenty of examples of people who looked good to me and to other faculty interviewers, people who seemed warm, spontaneous, thoughtful, and courteous, but then showed their true colors to the secretary in the residency office.

There are no detailed specifications for the ideal candidate, but I favor people who are more than just talented on paper, who are human beings with breadth of experience and maturity. In medicine, as in other professions, we want people to be just like us or like what we think we are. If we happen to be good doctors, that's good. There's a tendency to proselytize about one's field because it makes one feel good about oneself. We naturally try to justify what we're doing.

When all is said and done, we haven't turned out anyone about whom I feel uneasy. Two people had major problems with a certain aspect of internal medicine: in the ICU they were anxious and had trouble making important decisions quickly. One went into endocrinology and the other went into liaison consultative medicine with psychiatry. Both will be excellent in their specialties, but I'm glad they didn't go into acute care fields.

When you enter our program, you're heading toward becoming either a general internist or a specialist within internal medicine. The major subspecialty fields include infectious diseases, gastroenterology, rheumatology, cardiology, pulmonary medicine, critical care medicine, endocrinology, nephrology, and hematology-oncology. Most people decide about a subspecialty midway through their 3-year residency. A fellowship then adds 2 to 3 years of training, and then you can even superspecialize beyond that. For example, after a 3-year fellowship in cardiology, people commonly take an extra year to learn electrophysiology, angioplasty, or whatever. No one is obligated to make a decision about postresidency training during residency. It has become common for people to finish their residency training and not do a fellowship until after they have gone into practice (or worked in an emergency room, HMO, or urgent care center) for several years and begun to repay their medical school debt. Those who find it easiest to delay a fellowship are the ones who haven't had any delays from college through medical training. But I've found exceptions. Occasionally some people have the patience and the motivation to stick it out and not enter practice until they're in their mid- to late thirties.

Three specialty fellowships—pulmonary medicine, cardiology, and gastroenterology—are so competitive that they still have a matching system. The application is usually submitted a year and a half in advance, when you're at the early-to-middle segment of your second year of residency. You enter a matching process like the one that got you a residency. You learn the results in June of your second year, and then you have your third year of residency ahead of you before the fellowship starts. Most university fellowship programs give special consideration to their own residents. People who develop an interest in a superspecialty generally do so while they're doing the fellowship. As you narrow your field progressively, your relationships with patients become more episodic and less continuous and you become more technology-oriented.

For people who conclude during medical school that they want to work with adult patients but are uncertain about any specifics beyond that, I recommend an internal medicine internship as the first step. It's the most solid jumping off point for subsequent decisions, and after a year of medicine you can do almost anything, including psychiatry.

The issue of tension between being in a certain field of medicine and raising a family may influence your career choice. In some fields, such as emergency medicine, you can schedule your time predictably. In other fields, such as dermatology, you can look forward to few emergencies or unexpected hospital admissions. These fields attract people who expect to make a major time commitment to family life. I hasten to add that I know several individuals who are good and involved parents, and who are doing things like cardiology and even surgery. I don't know how they do it. I'm sure it's tough on either parent, but it's especially difficult if you're the mother because it requires great ingenuity and resourcefulness.

Training programs try to be accommodating and offer such help as parental leave policies. Our maternal leave policy allows for an 8-week absence. Our residents know that this is okay and that we expect colleagues in the residency program to be supportive. So that no one is taken by surprise and becomes hostile when called on to cover for a new parent, our maternal and paternal leave policy is published in the bylaws of house staff benefits. It is important to encourage paternal leave policy. We also try to help with the search for day care and schools. So far, no one has had to drop out because these problems became insurmountable, and our program is almost 40 percent female.

One issue regarding physicians that society keeps raising is their attitude toward financial gain. No residency candidate will come right out and tell us, "I owe $100,000 for my educational costs and I will have to take this into consideration in planning my future activities," but I know it lurks as a concern and I feel terrible about it. The technical specialties of medicine are overpaid and the cognitive ones underpaid. I hate the thought of losing good potential providers of primary and longitudinal care simply because those services are undervalued by the fee setters of our health care system. Unless changes are made, there will be a shortage in years to come.

Nothing is irrevocable when it comes to making a career choice; you can make a change at just about any phase of your working years. I have known people who were in midlife when they altered their direction in medicine and the change worked out well for them. Few people experience divine inspiration about what they are meant to do in medicine. You may identify someone like that in your medical school class and envy them for it, but for most of us, myself included, the reasons for our doing what we're doing are complex, subtle, and random. Medicine, regardless of the field, provides plenty of opportunities for a rewarding lifestyle, even if it is a close choice between plastic surgery and pediatric nephrology. Go with the flow and enjoy yourself.

Chapter 21

SURGERY

Dr. John Herrmann, a vascular surgeon, is a professor of surgery in the medical school of the University of Massachusetts Medical Center in Worcester. He was the program director of the surgical residency program for 8 years. He is now chair of the Division of Surgical Education in the Department of Surgery. He devotes about a third of his time to teaching and administration and the rest to clinical work.

John Herrmann, M.D., Vascular Surgery, Academic Medical Center

I think medicine is still one of the most rewarding careers in terms of personal satisfaction, and it's one of the most flexible careers. You can do almost anything you want within the broad spectrum of what constitutes the profession. I recommend a career in surgery, particularly for people with the appropriate characteristics. . . . After all these years, I'm still having a wonderful time.

Although my father was a pioneer in vascular surgery in this country, he tried to discourage me from going into medicine. Nevertheless, I ended up at Dartmouth College and Harvard Medical School. In my surgical clerkship I found that I liked vascular surgery, so that's been my clinical career; and now half of my professional life is devoted to medical teaching.

Over the years, I have talked with many medical students about their interests and career plans, but I still find it hard to define why some students go into surgery rather than medicine, pediatrics, or family practice. The considerations that attract people to medicine or other cognitive specialties are different from those that draw people to surgical or more mechanical, manipulative specialties. My father, an experienced metalworker, woodworker, plumber, and painter, taught me many skills, and I grew up mechanically inclined.

As a surgical residency program director, I find it hard to evaluate an applicant's manipulative skills because the recommendations tend to cover other attributes like intellect and clinical ability. I look for a student who plays a two-handed musical instrument, ties fishing flies, or does woodworking, and I explore the third-year surgical clerkship experience in relation to tying knots and using instruments. Most people can master the basics. We had one bright resident who compensated for blindness in one eye and is now a distinguished senior surgeon in a prominent clinic.

By and large, we base our acceptance on the usual criteria: academic performance, clinical skills, research potential, interpersonal relations, and personality traits. The latter two are probably the most important. Most medical school graduates are bright enough and can get by with reasonable clinical skills, but there can be personal flaws like not getting along with people, being lazy, trying to cover up mistakes by blaming others, or not getting the job done and saying they did. We have the most difficulty with residents who cannot get along with others.

I have had to counsel people out of surgery because of a character flaw. For me the one absolute disqualifier from any field of medicine is lack of integrity. You must be honest with yourself and everybody else. We can't accept the old European model where the professor ran the whole show and everyone adapted to the surgeon, who was technically gifted but irascible and difficult to work with. Surgery is no longer a one-man show; good results require team work.

One fading stereotype is that surgeons have only short relationships with patients. In the past, when surgical operations were often done as emergencies, the surgeon followed patients only briefly. Nowadays that may hold true for trauma surgeons, general surgeons who repair hernias and such, and often cardiac surgeons, but when you have a patient with a chronic condition like vascular disease, you are wedded to that patient for life. Especially with vascular disease we don't have medical angiologists to handle diagnostics and long-term conservative management, so a vascular surgeon does much of it.

If there ever was a surgical personality, it is far less differentiated today from the medical or pediatric personality. A good surgeon has defining attributes, but they are elusive and intangible. One characteristic that differentiates the surgeon is the ability to cope with the stress of making life-and-death decisions quickly and with limited information. Some people can't handle that emotionally. Internists have emergencies too, but more often than not they can go off and think about a problem, look it up in the library, or consult with colleagues. We try to weed out applicants who shy away from decision making or who shoot from the hip without the judgment, knowledge, or backup to make a good decision.

A hierarchical, physically demanding residency program brings out two problems. One is balancing independent decision making with appropriate prior consultation, and the other relates to personal time, the scarcity of which can be antithetical to a healthy lifestyle. We have resisted efforts to set fixed work hours for residents mainly because good patient care requires a resident to participate in all phases of clinical management. It is more of a calling than an on-the-job training program, and fixed time off is not good for education or patient care.

Surgeons often make poor family people. We have many divorces on the surgical service, and we try hard to ease the life of a surgical house officer by reducing hospital-imposed scut work like transporting patients, drawing bloods, and doing paper work. We are pioneers in the use of physician assistants and nurse practitioners to do tasks of limited educational value to residents.

That still leaves residents somewhat hospital-bound during training, but in the near future, even in surgery, about 70 percent of procedures will probably be done on an outpatient basis. Except in acute situations, most intellectual aspects, such as diagnosis, are done outside the hospital, and so a significant part of residency training is with ambulatory patients. But it is almost impossible to get a resident to go to the clinic if he has an operation that he would rather be doing. Training programs must provide meaningful pre- and posthospital experience. This is coming, pushed largely by managed care programs whereby patients enter the hospital worked up and virtually ready to climb on the operating table. One reason why medical students may have avoided primary care specialties in recent years is that they have seen patients mainly in the hospital and have missed the interaction between doctor and patient that occurs outside the hospital. When a resident works primarily in surgery and misses all the rest, it amounts to an inadequate educational experience—a technical exercise with exposure to only a small segment of medical care.

Because of the tight controls on bed utilization, patients who enter the hospital are sicker than before, and in academic medical centers especially, we work harder than ever. Until now, the demanding requirements of hospitalized patients had stimulated residency programs to expand enormously to provide cheap patient care. Now the programs are being trimmed and we still have to provide for educational programs along with everything else.

Many subdirections in surgery can provide a balanced family life. In subspecialties that make intense demands on time and physical energy, there are fewer women. A fair number of women are in surgical critical care; it's almost a shift type of situation. Some of the gender disparities may be due to discrimination, even today, but a lot of it is lifestyle. Very few women are in cardiothoracic surgery—it's tough to enter that club—but many other fields, such as ob/gyn, have almost been taken over by women even though the work takes a heavy toll on one's lifestyle. In plastic, breast, and endocrine surgery you can have much more control over your schedule, but general and trauma surgery are not very good for lifestyle.

As for who makes a better surgeon, one study of technical skills, spatial orientation, steadiness of hand, and so on suggested that in the beginning of their training women did better than men, but with time men improved more whereas women stayed about the same. Left-handers had considerable problems with technical skills. Instruments are designed for right-handed people and it's awkward for a right-handed person to assist a left-handed surgeon. We haven't had residents drop out because of being left-handed, but some women have dropped out because of being sensitive to biological time clocks or worrying about jeopardizing relationships with significant others. Yet we have had two married couples in the program at the same time, and residents have been married to residents in other programs, and all have made it through. This is less of an issue now than in days gone by.

To shift direction for a moment, the differences between medi-

cine and surgery have become blurred because many medical subspecialties are now procedure-oriented. Still, the way a medical student chooses between the two is often vague. He or she has limited
insight and sketchy information about life as a gastroenterologist or
a neurosurgeon, and may end up in a residency program that isn't
right. Most special disciplines, except for ob/gyn and ophthalmology, require at least 1 year of general surgical training, and this
period often gives people an idea of what kind of surgeon they want
to be or whether they really want to be a surgeon. We've had many
people start out in surgery and shift to anesthesiology, emergency
medicine, family practice, or pediatrics. It's tougher to go from medicine to surgery, but that has occurred.

It would be a big jump from internal medicine to cardiothoracic
surgery, but it's possible. More commonly it happens the other way,
perhaps because medical residencies are not quite as competitive as
surgical ones. Some surgical disciplines require 1 or 2 initial general
years whereas others, such as plastic, cardiothoracic, vascular, colon, rectal, and pediatric, require more, generally a full general surgical residency. With the latter group you can decide to apply as late
as the fourth year of general residency. Other surgical disciplines,
such as ophthalmology and orthopedic surgery, require a decision in
the second or third year of medical school, and for the life of me I
can't figure out how someone can make such a decision so early in
medical school. It usually involves a family connection, like your
father being an ophthalmologist.

Most of our applicants for general surgical training say that they
honestly don't know what they would eventually like to be, and
that's fine. We try to keep the first year of residency about the same
for the two classes of resident but we give the preliminary resident
a little more latitude in the choice of rotations. For instance, an
orthopedic surgeon might like to take a month of rheumatology or
radiology, whereas the categorical residents are in more of a lock-
step rotation.

You can take a stab at assessing your inner inclinations during a
general surgical training program. By your third or fourth year
you've seen enough of the surgical disciplines to have a good idea of
what each lifestyle is like, what type of work these people do, what
their stresses are, what their family life is like, what kind of people
they are, and what kind of patients they care for, and you can determine whether that's for you. Making decisions while you are in

medical school can be difficult. You need good advisors and opportunities to pick their brains. They should be in practice because the university academician is a rarefied breed, and most medical school graduates wind up in practice in community hospitals.

About 60 percent of residents go on to subspecialty training after completing a full course of general surgical training, leaving a smaller number headed for general surgery. It's becoming a needy specialty, and there's a big shortage coming along. Generalists do surgery of the abdomen; the skin and appendages, including breast; the endocrine, vascular, and gastrointestinal systems; and critical care and trauma interventions. Another problem relates to complicated procedures such as a Whipple operation for pancreatic cancer. Across the country there may be 2000 of these done a year, and only a quarter of them in teaching hospitals. A graduating chief resident in general surgery will have done one or none. Many of us feel that some of these complicated procedures should be done by a small group of highly trained specialists, perhaps on a regional basis. If I had to have my pancreas removed I'd prefer to go to someone who does the operation on a weekly basis rather than the surgeon who would be awfully good at taking care of my ruptured appendix. After basic training, a general surgeon should be permitted individualized training to specialize or at least have additional experience in, say, vascular or head and neck, as a general surgeon.

In the ongoing argument about the advantages and disadvantages of specialization, if you specialize too much, you get to know more and more about less and less. A specialist has a smaller body of knowledge to cope with, but because it goes deeper, the total amount of knowledge you have to master is about the same. The requirements in an urban community differ from those in a rural community where the general surgeon has to do orthopedics, urology, C sections, and otolaryngology. In New England we have numerous surgeons and specialists, and travel distances are small enough so people can get from one place to another without too much difficulty. However, rural areas require more generally oriented surgeons.

The generalists have more or less taken over laparoscopic work, probably out of pure self-preservation. The most common operation done in this country is cholecystectomy. If it is going to be done laparoscopically, general surgeons had better learn how to do it or they'll be out in the cold. Now they're even doing laparoscopic appendectomies, hernia repairs, colectomies, and so forth.

In this country most vascular surgery is done by general surgeons because there aren't enough vascular surgeons; we'd have to train twice the number we're currently training to meet the demand. As a result, the vascular surgeons tend to take care of the most complicated and difficult problems. I find myself seeing people whom nobody else wants to operate on because they're technically demanding, sick patients who are probably better managed in a university center by people who do that kind of work all the time. In the community hospital the average, less difficult vascular procedure is done by a general surgeon. Of course, as soon as a vascular surgeon comes into a community hospital, he takes over most of that work.

There's a great deal of maneuvering among groups to gain control over classes of patients and to exclude other doctors from doing this or that type of surgery. Vascular surgery is one area of controversy. Maxillofacial and head and neck surgery are others; so is breast surgery. Otolaryngology, plastics, and oral surgery also have their share of jockeying.

In the typical process of evolving into a surgeon, you take 5 years of general training and then probably an additional year or two of fellowship in a surgical specialty. Some general surgeons slip into a specialty not through a formal training plan but through a local medical manpower plan. Thus, someone in an academic institution may be asked to take over an area such as liver surgery and become expert in it. The developing expert may travel around, may take a fellowship with somebody doing interesting work in the area, and may set up a laboratory or experimental program on which to work.

If you finish surgical residency, become board-certified, and then find that you do not want to do surgery as a career, you can branch off into administration, work for a drug company, do site visits for joint commissions, and so on. If you decide early in training that you don't want to be a surgeon, then you can branch off into another field, such as anesthesiology, emergency medicine, internal medicine, pediatrics, or family practice, and get additional training to qualify in that area.

Many surgeons spend the early part of their career as busy clinical surgeons and later assume administrative or academic responsibilities, allowing their OR surgery to taper off and eventually disappear.

Part of the reason is that they never enjoyed it in the first place. Another part is burnout; they get tired of doing the same procedures day in and day out.

Medicine is changing. I don't know precisely where it's going, but it will be quite different in the 21st century. One major problem in our society is the cost of medical care. Because surgery is one of the more expensive types of care, the gatekeeper philosophy may shunt patients away from surgery for considerations based on reasons other than providing the best medical care.

Some wag once said that elective surgery is unnecessary surgery and therefore should not be done. You should wait for the hernia to become incarcerated or the ulcer to perforate before intervening. We are already seeing that thinking in cardiac surgery. Years ago we operated on "good"-risk cardiac patients; nowadays these patients are being treated nonsurgically with angioplasty or drugs and the surgical patients we see are much older and much poorer risks.

Where to do you draw the line in terms of cost–benefit ratio? I hate that term because I was trained to benefit the patients at all costs. However, society is saying that the cost is too great and that some decision making is necessary. The government would like the medical community to make the tough decisions and the medical community says it can't, government should do it. It's going to change the whole complex of medical care because medicine is now on a technological binge and we're doing things that certainly benefit a lot of patients, but at a high cost.

Studies have been done to evaluate the extent of unnecessary surgery and to explore whether an excess of surgeons has promoted it. This has been particularly studied in New England, where marked differences have been found from one area to another. It has been postulated that the presence of more surgeons leads to more surgery. One study done several years ago started with the premise that medical people would certainly not tolerate unnecessary surgery, and the investigators determined the incidence of surgical procedures among medical families vs. nonmedical families. The results showed that more procedures were done in the medical families.

As medicine evolves, most physicians would prefer that it remain as a cottage industry and that they continue with the independent decision making and self-sufficiency that go along with it. But we are being drawn rapidly into a much more industrialized method of delivering health care. Society is less willing to swallow the costs, which means that we must try to eliminate expensive procedures with no proven benefit. However, with procedures of proven benefit, other considerations come into the picture and the decisions become more difficult. Cardiac transplantation in a 45-year-old patient with cardiomyopathy who is the father of three children would seem to be cost-effective, whereas cardiac transplantation in an 80-year-old man who has failed three coronary bypasses probably is not justified. A big argument relates to bone marrow transplants for women with advanced breast cancer. There's no information that the procedure, which may cost hundreds of thousands of dollars, has any benefits, but some think it might and so women are clamoring for it. We need more well-designed clinical trials, but these are not easy to implement. When a doctor honestly believes that a procedure will benefit a patient, he or she is going to try to do it. After all, we are trained to be our patient's advocate. But the system is already intervening between the doctor and the decision. Most of the time we can adapt to it, but not always.

I have three children, none of whom is going into medicine. The closest they come is a daughter who is in a graduate masters program in nursing. I think medicine is still one of the most rewarding careers in terms of person satisfaction, and it's one of the most flexible careers. You can do almost anything you want within the broad spectrum of what constitutes the profession. I recommend a career in surgery, particularly for people with the appropriate characteristics. For most medical students surgery is a lot of fun—rolling up your sleeves, getting in there and doing things, and later seeing people get better. That is why students get interested in surgery, perhaps more so than they should. Early on it looks dynamic, but after not being home in 6 weeks to see their spouse and kids, students have second thoughts.

Today the tendency is definitely toward specialization regardless of what society is saying. Even if it means another year of training, surgical residents are looking for something to set themselves apart, to guarantee their self-sufficiency in the great wide world. I'm a specialist, but I spent many years practicing general surgery too. The advantage of being a general surgeon is that the spectrum of patients is broader; the advantage of being a specialist is that you're damn good at what you do and can hone it down. You can enjoy both. The advantage of academic medicine is that you wear lots of hats, and if you get tired of doing one thing you can do something else. The multitalented academician can no longer function as such. You cannot do a good job as an able researcher, a superb teacher, an effective administrator, and a top-notch clinician all at the same time, and so you specialize within the academic field. But again, there are many choices.

For a few years, medicine was looked at as a very financially rewarding field. If you liked science in college, you could go into clinical medicine, do research, make lots of money, and have a wonderful lifestyle. That has faded. You can probably make more money as a stockbroker than as a physician. The days of the type of remuneration that physicians got in the last generation are rapidly receding.

The problem of repaying loans for medical education will make a difference in the choice of medical disciplines. Nobody want to pay for educating medical students—not government, not third-party payers, not faculty. Who wants to pay to have a bunch of rich young kids get educated to be wealthy doctors? So the students come out with debts that make it tough for them to become primary care physicians; yet we need more of those. We ought to make the primary care specialties more rewarding, not just monetarily but also in terms of gratification and prestige. It's harder to be a good primary care physician than it is to be a specialist. Even I have do some primary care, and some of the more interesting problems that I run into are the ones for which I don't have a ready answer and have to consult the literature. After all these years, I'm still having a wonderful time.

Chapter 22

PSYCHIATRY

Dr. Paul Barreira is an associate professor of psychiatry in the school of medicine at the University of Massachusetts Medical Center in Worcester. He is also director of the Psychiatry Residency Training Program.

Paul Barreira, M.D., Psychiatry, Academic Medical Center

In my 8 years as director of the residency training program we admitted a number of people who, in retrospect, should not have gone into psychiatry. A couple whom I counseled out eventually went into internal medicine. In several instances I thought they did not have the temperament for clinical work of any kind and I suggested fields not involving face-to-face patient work such as radiology or anesthesiology. There are some good fields where such people can put their intellectual capacities to use without having the emotional strain of patient contact.

I'm the only person in my family who went to college. I'm from a Portuguese community in Somerville, Massachusetts. When I was a child we moved to Cleveland where I went to a public high school. Then I started out at Purdue University because I was interested in math and science. Very soon thereafter, I transferred to Boston College to major in philosophy and premed. I wanted to become a psychiatrist or a clinical psychologist. In my senior year of college, I left before graduating and joined the Jesuits to become a priest. I stayed in for 10 years, 2 of which I spent in a seminary in the Berkshires. I went through Georgetown Medical School and started training in psychiatry while still a Jesuit.

My medical school years confirmed that I enjoyed medicine and psychiatry. To solidify my identity as a physician, I completed a medical internship at the Hartford Hospital in Connecticut before starting my psychiatry residency. During medical school, at the suggestion of the psychiatry chairman, I did an outside elective at the Beth Israel Hospital in Boston, where I liked the people I met, especially the residents and the faculty. I elected to go there for residency training because I was interested in psychoanalysis and they had a strong analytic faculty. In the early 1970s, the analytic psychotherapy school was still prominent in academic centers in this country, which influenced me in medical school. In addition, my earlier reading had been in philosophy, and much of Freud is similar to it.

I started with a general residency in psychiatry. Because the residency had a distinct analytic emphasis, it was expected that after 3 to 4 years I would join a psychoanalytic institute for 7 to 9 years. Furthermore, I had to complete two "controlled analyses" by seeing two patients as a supervised trainee. In my first year in residency I started my own analysis with a psychiatrist who was then the dean of the Analytic Institute in Boston. He assumed that eventually I would join the Institute. But during my residency, I discovered neuropsychiatry, neuroendocrinology, and the biological theory of mood and psychotic disorders. I also came to appreciate alternative psychological models such as family systems theory and cognitive behavior models.

My options for a career decision expanded tremendously. For a couple of years I stayed at Beth Israel and ran a psychiatric service within the internal medicine primary care clinic. Then I took a clinical research fellowship at McLean Hospital to study mood disorders with emphasis on the pharmacologic treatment of mania and depression. Although I did my own personal analysis, I didn't do a practice analysis. Today I make use of what I learned from all of the factions. I try to use the insights provided by the analytic approach as well as those arising from the biological framework.

Psychiatry has always needed science to make it respectable in medicine, and now it seems to be moving in the direction of the brain as the mechanism by which the body works and divorcing itself from the approach to patients as whole organisms, with personal histories, feelings, and lives connected to their families and to their social, spiritual, and professional communities. In contrast, my primary care friends are emphasizing medical interviewing, feeling connected to patients, and appreciating other aspects of their lives. It's a dialectic that gets played over and over again. Each generation of physicians faces the challenge of how much of the tremendous body of knowledge and technology they can integrate into what is essentially an interpersonal event. The pendulum has swung now more toward the technical, due perhaps to economic forces, but we should listen to the patients and not necessarily the economists.

The medical students who seem interested in psychiatry appear to be curious about why people act the way they do and their curiosity goes beyond motivational theory to questions about what's going on in the brain. What happens in the brain that makes people have hallucinatory experiences? Why do people suddenly experience terribly depressed moods that are totally foreign to them and that seem to come from nowhere? What does this tell us about the relation between mind and brain? Those questions get the bright students terribly excited about psychiatry, the ones who are not intimidated by the seriousness of chronic mental illness or by the blurred boundaries in psychiatry and neurology, psychiatry and psychology, and psychiatry and medicine. They're the ones who do well in residency.

Most psychiatrists still act as clinicians doing one-to-one work, but now they seem to be doing it in group settings. Rather than having an office and seeing one patient for 50 minutes, they're more likely to be part of a broader medical practice that combines different models of treatment. They'll do short-term talking therapy, prescribe medication, and do consults. Yet another way to divide the pie is by the setting. For example, some people like inpatient psychiatry. By the fourth year of training, general psychiatry residents have begun to identify what they do and don't like in psychiatry and what they do and don't do well. During the residency they experience the different settings in which one might practice psychiatry. Our residents do inpatient psychiatry in the university unit and the state hospital unit, and they do consultation liaison psychiatry on medical and surgical wards.

It's asking a lot of students to understand themselves by the third year of medical school when they have to choose a specialty. One of my best residents is graduating from a general adult psychiatry program this year. As a senior in medical school, he came to me at the end of the residency interviewing season and said, "You know, I already have an ophthalmology residency lined up, and they're hard to come by. But it just doesn't sit well with me." He liked his psychiatry rotations but got caught up in the scientific and technical aspects of ophthalmology. Having the position in hand so early forced him to think about whether he really wanted the field. If he hadn't been accepted, he probably would still be lusting after the ophthalmology residency. Once he had it, though, suddenly he wasn't all that sure. He did a last minute extra rotation in psychiatry in his senior year, after which he applied and was accepted. He couldn't have pulled an eleventh hour switch like that from psychiatry to ophthalmology.

My impression is that many students are somewhat interested in psychiatry but are hesitant about it. They start off in another field and then later come to psychiatry. I recruited some terrific resident candidates after they had been through a year of two of medicine. I know several surgeons who came into psychiatry. One was my classmate when I was resident.

During the first 3 years out of medical school one can still make shifts at little cost in terms of years of training. After 3 years it becomes more difficult. Every year I see one or two people who have been in practice in another field and have quit to enter psychiatry. Generally they do well. The ones about whom I have questions are bright people who go immediately from one residency to another, or do 2 years in one residency, don't complete it, and go into another residency. They're not settling down into something. It doesn't happen very often but you see it. Their prognosis is poor. They appear chronically unhappy and never commit to anything.

In my 8 years as director of the residency training program we admitted a number of people who, in retrospect, should not have gone into psychiatry. A couple whom I counseled out eventually went into internal medicine. In several instances I thought they did not have the temperament for clinical work of any kind and I suggested fields not involving face-to-face patient work such as radiology or anesthesiology. There are some good fields where such people can put their intellectual capacities to use without having the emotional strain of patient contact.

The question of whether people go into psychiatry in search of self-help is fascinating because in the 1960s and early 1970s it was the norm that people training for psychiatry would undergo treatment. There was the sense that if you wanted to help people you had to understand your own problems and know what it meant to be in treatment. That's less true now. Many students are attracted to psychiatry because family members, friends, and maybe even they themselves have been helped through emotional distress by clinical care. I worry about residency applicants who exhibit too strong a connection between their needing help and thinking that going into psychiatry is a way of getting it.

Concerning my own training, after my research fellowship at McLean I came here as the residency training director in general adult psychiatry. At some expense to my academic career, I've remained a generalist and have not developed the expertise that fosters academic productivity. I work especially well with patients with mood disorders, psychotic illnesses, and the like, but I refuse to be pigeonholed as a psychopharmacologist or psychotherapist. I use whatever I can to help people with such conditions.

The issue of specialization affects psychiatry as much as any other field. We're moving toward increasing the number of specialty boards in psychiatry, which has prompted a lively national debate about whether we should be required to have special tracking with board certification—as now occurs with child and adolescent psychiatry—to go into such areas as substance abuse, consultation liaison, geriatric psychiatry, and forensic psychiatry. Part of what drives it is economics; people strive for a niche with sufficient market share. In academic centers young doctors want to establish themselves as having expertise in an area that will enable them to climb the academic ladder. Those are two of the forces for specialization, and I'm not convinced they lead to better medical care for patients.

As for a solution, we need to distinguish between what's necessary in academe and what's needed for good patient care outside the training centers. The linchpin of medical care is the general practitioner, the doctor who sees the patient first. That position must be given enormous prestige and self-esteem in the delivery of health care. To accomplish that, we have to legislate it. The income discrepancies among medical fields must be reduced and the public has to learn what good medical care is. People must be willing to see the generalist as a central figure in health care—the doctor on whom they count for the first opinion about their complaint and the doctor they trust to know when someone else should be consulted. The generalist will take care of about 80 percent of what bothers them for most of their life. By not accepting this system the public is driving the push toward specialization. No matter what, we need general psychiatrists, but their number is diminishing and no one clearly understands why.

Some practitioners get tired emotionally and vary aspects of their practice. Instead of working 40 hours a week seeing one patient after another, they may change to half-time work at a community health center where they may supervise other physicians, provide consultations, teach, and see patients in a different setting. I think people who start out working that way are happier and don't burn out as much.

Medical students considering a career in psychiatry should talk with a faculty member in the department. Faculty universally respond positively to a student's interest in their field. It will help students to learn what the faculty do, what they think about, what their practices are like, what kind of research is going on in their field, what new drugs are used, and the like. A 6-week clerkship is often too short a time to become familiar with the field, and even a course in behavioral sciences in the basic science years is not enough.

As for the people with whom I work every day, I don't like them as "stereotypes" but I like them as individuals. I respect their professional skills and their attitudes about medicine, life, and people. I'm in psychiatry because I like the people and because the value system is synergistic with mine.

In sizing up our residency candidates I look for people who, by their way of relating to me and by the stories they tell me, appear emotionally mature, curious, capable of living with uncertainty, and tolerant of affect. If a patient cries and looks sad, you tolerate it, sit with the person, and help him or her see what it's all about. So I look for people who don't feel that every time they see a signal from a patient they have to do something. I can't tell all that from an interview. I like to have recommendations from surgeons, internists, and pediatricians, in addition to psychiatrists. Such recommendations carry enormous weight. I want to know that somebody is viewed as a competent physician. To the extent that there are universal qualities that make for good physicians (such as being smart, being sensitive to one's own needs and to those of patients, having reasonable expectations of oneself, knowing how to evaluate and organize data, and being compassionate), I want to know what the teachers think about a student. For example, it means a lot when a pediatrician says that a student would make a terrific pediatrician, relates well to kids and their families, and understands medical science.

I don't react well to people who have made premature closure about what they're going to do in psychiatry. I prefer a student who wants first to find out what general psychiatry is about and whose mind is open to the different models in use today. If only one model had the truth, there wouldn't be this cacophony of conceptual models. When residents appear to be going off prematurely in one direction, I make sure they are exposed to other directions. For example, if an applicant says he or she wants to be a Jungian analyst, I am not inclined to recruit that person because his or her mind seems too closed.

We don't have many late entrants into psychiatry. When one does come along, I look for the motives for the change. The most positive motive is that the applicant likes certain aspects of his or her practice, can't do them enough, and perceives psychiatry as a way of doing more. An example would be the practitioner who says, "I find myself talking with patients about their emotional problems or their family interactions, but I never have enough time for that and end up referring them to someone else. I'd rather be the one they're being referred to." I also try to get a sense of what impact the change will have on the applicant's family or significant others and whether the person has considered what it will be like to take call every third night and to make do with a resident's income. I ask them how they think they will react to reporting to younger people and to being a student again.

My 11-year-old daughter wants to go to Yale Drama School. I have no idea whether she will someday consider psychiatry. If she were to ask me about going into medicine and showed a definite interest, I would certainly encourage her to enter the field. I think she sees me as being very happy with what I'm doing, and she's right!

Chapter 23

PEDIATRICS

Dr. Evan Charney is the chairman of the Department of Pediatrics in the medical school and the executive director of the Children's Medical Center at the University of Massachusetts Medical Center in Worcester. During his first year as chair of pediatrics, he directed the residency training program. He is also chairman of the Residency Review Committee for Pediatrics of the Accreditation Council for Graduate Medical Education. What professional time he has left over from administration he devotes to teaching, patient care, and research.

Evan Charney, M.D., General Pediatrics, Academic Medical Center

People go into pediatrics because of a love for children and a commitment to advocate for their welfare. The field is exciting and I have never once regretted my choice. I am absolutely enjoying it. As for whether I will ever return to art, that's another matter.

I was born and raised in the Bronx and went to the High School of Music and Art where I majored in art. Although I had decided at age 7 to become an artist, when I saw how talented other students were I settled for art as an avocation. I went on to Cornell University and majored in psychology. Until my senior year, I thought about going into experimental psychology or high school teaching; then I decided to go into medicine. The idea of dealing only with visual perceptions in a rat, or even a human being, seemed dull. A career without regular interaction with people, particularly in a helping way, appeared inappropriate. Although no one in my family had been a physician, I had once spent a few days with a surgeon and was impressed by how much he loved what he did. I very much wanted to do something that I would love and that would be a calling.

During college I was in the ROTC (the Korean War was on) and when I graduated, I went into the army for 2 years as a tank repair officer. Although I'd barely taken the requisite courses, I applied for medical school while still in the army. Albert Einstein, which was a new school at the time, accepted me into its second class.

I did well during the first 2 years but saw no patients at all. The school's emphasis was heavily on basic research. The chairman of medicine was a great investigator who had created a superb research department, but he appeared uneasy with patients. After the medicine clerkship I began to question my choice of a career. I thought, "If this is medicine, it's not for me." Then I rotated into pediatrics and immediately felt at home because of the people and the discipline.

To be a pediatrician, you must love children, and I do. I felt comfortable, and I saw in the pediatricians the kind of person I thought I could be. They were superb clinician–teachers and wonderful role models. They also had a broad view of medicine and were dedicated advocates for the welfare of children. They thought beyond the four walls of the hospital. It all seemed right, and I felt that at last I knew who I was. Of course, had I been exposed to a different sort of department of medicine, I might have become an internist.

Time, place, and people have a lot to do with the decision of what field to enter. Most students look on the decision as an analytic process that involves balancing assets against liabilities, but in the end it's a gut decision. Listing positives and negatives is helpful, but feelings count for more. Besides, there is no correct decision; a person can be happy in many fields.

By decision-making time some students are reasonably insightful about their personal makeup and some are not. Most medical schools, including ours, could do a better job of helping students through the decision making. Starting in the first year and continuing through the 4 years, faculty in each of the disciplines ought to share their thoughts about the nature of their field and its relation to professional and personal life. Instead, we assume that somehow the third-year clinical clerkship is a valid mirror of what a field is, and yet that's not strictly correct. Also, for role models a student looks to residents because they're younger and more accessible than faculty, and that's appropriate, but nobody remains a resident for life. If we faculty were more helpful, students would be better prepared to make the decision about the basic cut: medicine, surgery, primary care, subspecialty, and so on. On the matter of whether fields have defined personality types, some of the truisms are valid generalizations, but for individuals there can be great variation.

In my third year, I considered all of the alternatives but pediatrics won out. I left open the question of where I was heading within pediatrics and even now I'm working on that. For my residency I went to the University of Rochester. I thought they had a breadth of faculty there, but that was laughable because they had only about five people in pediatrics. They were strong in some subspecialty disciplines that were emerging, and it was appealing to get out of New York City and try a different community. In addition, the department and the school had a strong reputation for scholarship. Incidentally, I had been married not too much earlier and we had a 2-month-old baby.

It was during the residency years that my next step emerged. By the last year I had focused on hematology and oncology. But that was a different era in oncology, and in my last year all of the children I cared for died and the faculty person became clinically depressed. I had been planning to apply for a fellowship in oncology and hematology but concluded that I couldn't do the work. I determined that I would like to practice, but I loved being at a referral center and heard about a unique program in a rural New Jersey community populated by old-style general practitioners. The regional hospital had set up a geographic full-time group of subspecialists to serve as a referral source and to care for the children with complex illnesses that required hospitalization. There were academic ties to Columbia and Cornell. That program was enormously appealing. They suggested that since I was coming directly from a residency, I might want to get more depth in one field or another before joining them. So I took a fellowship in what came to be family medicine at the Children's Hospital in Boston and worked in adolescent medicine, then a nascent field.

That experience sharpened my general diagnostic skills and brought me under the influence of Robert Haggerty, the fellowship director. He epitomized everything that I loved about pediatrics and he became my mentor and role model. During the fellowship, Haggerty was made chairman of pediatrics at the University of Rochester and asked me to join him there. I left New Jersey and went with him to direct the ambulatory and community programs. I didn't have a clear idea of what that meant, but the move changed my career.

Those were exciting days in the 1960s. We developed one of the first neighborhood health centers in the United States; we established nurse practitioner training programs for pediatrics; and we developed a collaborative research program with community practitioners. I directed all of those projects, which made for heady times because a new field of primary care was coming into being. I worked at it for 12 years at Rochester and then I wanted to try something else in a community-based program. I elected to take on a large but not too well-developed community program out of the Sinai Hospital in Baltimore, a Johns Hopkins affiliate, and to try out some ideas in medical education and service to the community. I spent the next 12 years there.

At Sinai we developed a primary care program for a low-income, largely black community. We eliminated the entire clinic and opened a group practice that made the quality of care probably the best or close to it that one could receive in Baltimore, and we developed a training program for primary care generalists. It is still going strong, like the one at Rochester. Then I became the chairman here.

The current question in medicine—where have all the generalists gone?—is less of a problem in pediatrics than in adult practice. Unlike family practice and internal medicine, in pediatrics there has not been a drop in student interest. Between 8 and 10 percent of U.S. graduates have continued to select pediatrics for the past decade. That's been sustained by the increase in the proportion of women in medical school classes; women choose pediatrics disproportionately in relation to family and internal medicine. I think that women have a sensitivity, either by nature or nurture, to the needs of children and feel comfortable with children's issues. Furthermore, they are welcomed in pediatrics. But for that trend, we probably would have had a reduction in people going into our field.

Why are fewer people choosing generalist fields? There's no single, simple answer. Over the years, the devaluation of primary care has taken a gradual toll. Students are rarely exposed to primary care practitioners who are satisfied with what they do and most of their role models are subspecialists based in tertiary care centers.

With an average student indebtedness of $50,000–$100,000, finances enter into the choice of a career direction. Pediatrics, along with family practice and psychiatry, is one of the lowest reimbursed fields, not that I think pediatricians are underpaid. Also, students now want to combine the practice of medicine with a reasonable family life and enjoy themselves, whereas 50 years ago doctors practiced their calling 70 hours a week. Subspecialty fields like radiology, ophthalmology, and dermatology offer higher reimbursement and enable physicians to work less hard if they so choose. However, from this lifestyle point of view, I think pediatrics is a satisfying career in the current group practice model. Group practices, HMOs, and other large aggregations of physicians allow for a lifestyle that is consonant with a good family life and may be even easier than in academic pediatrics.

I have been selecting residents in pediatrics for 17 years. All pediatricians, whether they end up as molecular subspecialists or rural primary care doctors, take the same 3-year general pediatric residency. There is plenty of time to decide your next step. You should look for a broadly based generalist program. Obtaining a fellowship is less competitive than matching into a residency, which is less competitive than entering medical school. So, with some exceptions, if you're good, you can get into fellowship training from any accredited pediatric residency.

The real question is how to design the next step after general residency. In some ways, it's a miniversion of the selection of the field itself during medical school. To make an informed choice, you need to select a residency that provides exposure both to primary care practice and to subspecialty pediatrics. Training programs vary greatly in that regard; of the 215 accredited pediatric residency programs in the United States, about half are community programs and half are university programs. In general, university programs and some community programs have a sufficient breadth of subspecialists so that residents can observe the practices and lifestyles of those people but it is not as easy to get a valid exposure to community-based practice.

In our program residents work in community-based practices 1 or 2 half days a week for their entire 3 years and see real life practice. They become a junior partner in a practice and have about 100–200 patients of their own whom they see on a regular basis and for whom they provide care. Virtually without exception the patients welcome the arrangement. The supervising practitioners go through a formal educational program in our department to learn how to teach in this setting.

If you reach the end of medical school still not sure about your generalist or specialist orientation, pediatrics affords you an opportunity to continue to keep that option open, whereas family medicine does not. By definition family practice physicians are not specialists. That's the strength of the field and I have a lot of respect for family medicine. However, it would be much harder to go into cardiology after 3 years of training in family medicine, than after 3 years of training in general pediatrics.

In contrast to family practice, pediatrics is more rooted in the joy of working with children and affords greater opportunity to go more deeply into their diseases, problems, and health issues. You have to choose your focus—children or the entire family. Even now, in departments of medicine and pediatrics, feelings flourish that family practice requires less capability and skill. I do not subscribe to that view.

Some medically sophisticated patients feel that because a primary care doctor has to cover such a wide range of clinical problems, his or her ability to handle less obvious situations diminishes; hence it is better to have a subspecialist take on their primary care needs. There's some validity to that, but it involves a tradeoff. Certainly a good subspecialist is better than a poor generalist. The optimum model is to be under the care of a good generalist who works well with subspecialists and who uses them appropriately for consultation and referral. A child with a chronic condition will get better care from both than from either one alone. There are exceptions. The child with leukemia needs such specialized care that virtually all of the care will be given by a pediatric oncologist. Yet the broader needs of that child for other health issues (immunization, school performance, and the impact of the disease on siblings) are often foremost in the mind of the generalist and may be less so for the subspecialist. When one has to choose experimental treatments the generalist who serves as advocate for the welfare of the patient has an important role to play in helping the family to reach the best decision for them.

I do not feel in any way that the specialist is less humane, less caring, or less competent. We're talking about breadth of responsibility, not depth of commitment. It is true that sometimes a specialist whose skill is especially uncommon and in high demand may have less time to sit and interact with the patient and may therefore convey an aura of indifference. What is becoming common in pediatric specialty care—and oncology is a good example, although not the exclusive one—is to provide a team of professionals. In all of our specialty divisions we have teams that include nurse practitioners, social workers, and others who have a broad vision of the patient's social and psychological needs. Many programs, such as rehabilitation services for children, can be done across disciplinary lines, and the development of children's centers fosters the capacity to work across these lines.

If at the end of 3 years of a residency in general pediatrics you want to practice primary care, you should have acquired enough skills during your training to step into practice without a fellowship. We could do better in preparing people to go directly into practice. If you are heading into subspecialty training, then you have 3 additional fellowship years ahead of you. There are also general academic fellowships that prepare people to be teachers and researchers in general academic pediatrics.

It used to be universally true that if you wanted to teach you aimed at a career based in a medical school setting. However, along with the greater emphasis on preparing generalists is an evolving need to include community-based practicing faculty as teachers; and so in many places you can have a strong role as a teacher for medical students and residents while working in a community-based practice.

The choice between generalist and specialist is mostly made by happenstance. For the generalist, the child and its family is the center of professional life; the diseases come and go but the patient stays. For the specialist, the disease stays and the patients come and go. That's a generalization, but I think that if you are fascinated by the disease or the organ, and if you find that intellectually stimulating and emotionally satisfying, you probably would enjoy a career as a specialist. If you gravitate toward watching children and families grow and change, and toward helping them cope with life's medical and other stresses, then primary care is the field for you.

In pediatrics, unlike internal medicine, the vast majority of sub-specialists are based in a tertiary care hospital, and that often means an academic medical center. About 85 percent of pediatricians are generalists and about 15 percent are subspecialists. Subspecialties in pediatrics are similar to those in internal medicine: hematology, oncology, neurology, gastroenterology, critical care, and the like. In addition, there are two age-specific specialties: neonatology and adolescent medicine. New pediatric specialties are percolating—pediatric emergency medicine, for example.

In choosing pediatric residents, the warning signs are much like those for medicine in general, and they relate to emotional instability. That is probably the most serious problem and often the most difficult to detect. We are rarely informed about serious emotional problems that a medical student may have had. It's a complex issue involving the right to privacy, but it could lead to disaster.

In a stable person there is still the issue of fit. As with most other disciplines, the vast majority of people who enter pediatric training complete it and then practice in the field. That is due partly to good choices and partly to the fact that many medical students are talented people who can do many jobs well. Particularly important is having a real love for children and a joy in working with them. If an applicant doesn't feel that, then he or she doesn't belong in pediatrics. Why someone will be drawn to the concerns of children probably falls under the mystery of life. A lot of it is based on past experience in working with children—in summer camp, in slum settings, or in foreign lands. People who have not managed to interact with children during the first 26 years of their life are not likely to find their way into pediatrics.

Pediatrics can accommodate a broad range of interests and talents from the molecular geneticist to the rural practitioner. You can find happiness in any one of a number of career paths within pediatrics and there isn't just one personality type that fits. Not many people leave pediatric training but those who do have a variety of reasons. Some discover that they like a more surgical or more instrumental kind of work such as anesthesiology, where personal interactions are less intense and easier to cope with. Others, a smaller number, go into such fields as radiology and pathology to move away from patients altogether. And there are some who are so caught up in the emotional problems of children that they cannot stand to deal with medical illness and move instead into child psychiatry. Some of these individuals do brilliantly well. Incidentally, I feel that anyone who is headed into child psychiatry should start with a year of general pediatrics. It isn't required, but it should be.

For the right person pediatrics is a wonderful life. I'm optimistic about its future, both the primary care and the subspecialty segments. During the next 10 years there will be major evolutions in primary care and subspecialty pediatrics. Molecular genetics is going to revolutionize the practice of pediatrics. What that means and how it will come about, I haven't the faintest idea. In addition to installing genes to correct inherited defects, there is the daunting vision of being able to ascertain the genetic heritage of a newborn infant—what it's likely to suffer from later on and what it's not likely to encounter. It may not be all positive, but it will be possible.

Another issue is neonatal medicine, where we run head on into the economics of health care. The present balance is clearly out of whack. It isn't that the neonatologists are doing wrong; they're doing the job assigned to them and doing it well. More and more of the children they save face an improved prognosis. The progress is steady and impressive, but we are pushing the limit of viable size. An equally important task is preventing these small births. That's the nation's job, but pediatricians have a role to play. Though I haven't mentioned it yet, one of the things that distinguishes pediatrics from every other field of medicine is our motto that we "advocate for the welfare of children." Our aspiration to do that distinguishes us from surgery, internal medicine, and even family medicine, and pediatrics attracts students with that kind of social commitment.

Within pediatrics some fields have distinctive characteristics. neonatology, critical care medicine, and emergency medicine are characterized by more technology and look more like the surgical specialties.

For some reason, this brings me to the subject of midlife course correction. That's a challenge for medicine as a whole, particularly for primary care. In academic medicine or in specialties it is not uncommon for a doctor to move through career changes, but until recently it has been harder for a primary care practitioner to do that. We need to design changes that will make career moves easier for the practicing pediatrician, the family practitioner, or the internist.

First, we must reassure them that midlife changes are not wrong, not walking away from an obligation. Within pediatrics there are specialty areas that could benefit greatly from people with 5 or 10 years of seasoning. With handicapped children, behavioral pediatrics, and school health, we could benefit from someone with a deep background and a wealth of experience in primary care practice. Some retraining or additional training may be needed, and a process ought to be established to facilitate such moves. A growing special area involves working with children who are victims of physical and sexual abuse. It, too, requires special training.

People go into pediatrics because of a love for children and a commitment to advocate for their welfare. The field is exciting and I have never once regretted my choice. I am absolutely enjoying it. As for whether I will ever return to art, that's another matter.

Part Four

NATIONAL HEALTH POLICY— PARTICIPATING PHYSICIANS

When it comes to health policy, as Jimmy Durante used to say, "everybody wants to get into the act." Because the questions related to health care are so important to all of us, it is appropriate for "everybody" to get into the act, physicians included, perhaps even more so.

Some doctors go beyond talking and debating. They jump into the action and contribute much of their time, concern, and commitment. Occasionally their involvement leads to personal sacrifice or harsh public treatment. The stories in this section describe three doctors who are motivated to play a role in changing pivotal features of the country's health care system. Their common denominator is a desire to improve medical care for people.

Dr. Howard Dean, a general internist, became the governor of a state where he is now trying to implement a number of fundamental ideas for enhancing various aspects of the health care of his constituents. Dr. Joycelyn Elders left academic pediatric endocrinology to become a health care administrator, first in Arkansas as head of the state's health department and then in Washington as Surgeon General of the U.S. Public Health Service. After a term of service in which she spoke out frankly about what she regards as common sense approaches to our major health care problems, especially those related to children, in December 1994, she resigned from her position as Surgeon General and returned to Arkansas. Dr. Arnold Relman, a nephrologist and a medical educator, spent a decade as editor-in-chief of the *New England Journal of Medicine*, an international forum for, among other things, the exchange of ideas about policy questions related to health care.

I thought it would be interesting to medical students and residents who will be entering the world of medicine after some far-reaching changes have modified basic aspects of their professional lives to read about the factors and circumstances that led these three physicians to their involvement in policy issues and to learn what they think ought to be done in the time ahead to modify our national approaches to medical care.

Chapter 24

STATE GOVERNOR

Dr. Howard Dean practiced internal medicine in Vermont, ran for the state legislature, later became lieutenant governor, and then took over the governorship when the incumbent governor died. At the time of this interview, Dr. Dean was running for his first term as an elected governor, a race he went on to win.

Howard Dean, M.D., Internist and Governor of Vermont

Medical education is all about accomplishing things for other people and helping them. There are ways to help people as a doctor other than by seeing them in the office.

I grew up in East Hampton, Long Island. My father was a stockbroker. I went to the St. George School in Newport, Rhode Island, and then to Yale where I studied political science. In high school I always liked science too. After Yale, I went to Aspen to ski. To support myself, I washed dishes, poured concrete, and took other similar jobs, but eventually I decided that I wanted a real challenge, and that decision came down to three choices: teaching, for which I was qualified by my studies at Yale; practicing medicine, toward which I had some draw because an uncle was an internist; and selling stocks and bonds, like my father.

I went into the brokerage business in New York City and, after a year and a half, found that I didn't like the job or the place. A friend had gone back to school to prepare for applying to medical school, and I decided to do the same. I took a biology course at Columbia's night school and volunteered in the emergency room at St. Vincent's Hospital. I did well in the course, and after 5 months I quit work, moved into my parents' place in New York City, and attended Columbia full time to satisfy premedical requirements. By then I was sure that I wanted to become a doctor.

After about a year, I was accepted into a 3-year program at the Albert Einstein Medical School. After medical school, I came up here to Vermont to do my residency training. I chose internal medicine because it had been my favorite clerkship. Other areas I considered were psychiatry and surgery. I rejected psychiatry because I didn't think I could spend 8 hours a day listening to people's problems, but ironically that is frequently what a governor does. As for surgery, I didn't want to be wedded to a hospital. Internal medicine was challenging, intellectual, and enjoyable.

Toward the end of my internship, I made the decision to practice general internal medicine and not do a specialty after my residency. I had met my wife Judy at Einstein. She, too, chose to go into internal medicine and is board-eligible in hematology and oncology. She's from New York as well, but we ended up in Vermont because I have had long connections with this state. My brother went to the University of Vermont and I've been coming here to ski since 1967. Vermont's medical school had an excellent ambulatory care track, and I put it high up on my list of choices for hospital training. Judy came up here after I made my decision.

In the second year of my residency I became very involved in politics. The state senator, who was running Jimmy Carter's re-election campaign, lived near us and became a good friend. I worked as a Carter campaign volunteer while I was a resident.

After the third year of residency, I joined a two-person practice, taking over for an older physician. When my wife finished her residency, she did a year of hematology at McGill, finished off 2 more years in oncology at the University of Vermont, and then joined our practice.

I had often thought about a political career. There's a lot to be done in this country and in the world in general to improve life for people, and I think the political arena is where you get many of those things done. Most of that feeling stems from an inner drive. However, some of it also comes from my parents even though they're Republicans and I'm a Democrat. When I was in college in the 1960s and 1970s, I was opposed to the war and had much more in common with the Democrats than with the Republicans.

As a result of the Carter campaign, I went to the 1980 convention in New York as a Vermont delegate and got to know a lot of people. I pretty much decided that at some point I was going to run for office. Even when I interviewed for entry into the practice, I made it clear to my future partner that I would be running for the legislature one day. The legislature is a part-time job here, meeting only part of the year, and then only on Tuesday, Wednesday, Thursday, and half of Friday.

After I was elected, I kept a full practice going. I would go back home and have evening office hours on Tuesday, Wednesday, and Thursday, and then work half of Friday, half of Saturday, and all of Monday. Some of the older patients felt that if I wasn't right there, I wasn't anywhere, but the reality is that in a medical practice you're covered for emergencies—and there aren't that many of them. Usually, it creates no big problem to come in at 5 o'clock in the afternoon instead of 10 o'clock in the morning; in fact, several of the working people preferred the evening office hours.

As a family we cope with my schedule rather well. Since my wife is very busy too, we have had to work hard at it. When I became governor we decided that we finally needed some live-in help. Before that, the lieutenant governor job was also part time, so for most of my time in that position I was able to keep up with my practice. We had good babysitters and the children didn't need chauffeuring when they were young. Mostly, they needed good child care, which we had. We live in Burlington, about 40 minutes away from the capitol. The drive back and forth was part of my life only during the legislature sessions, which run from the first week in January to mid-May.

Since my time in medical school, I have believed that we ought to have national health insurance. During my senior clerkships, I spent a month in Washington traipsing around the Hill and following what was going on in relation to national health insurance. As I now have the unusual opportunity of seeing my ideas implemented in an entire state, I think I'm incorporating some of these new ideas with long overdue ones into our state's program for health care reform. It's a complicated matter and is given to oversimplification by politicians for their own ends. In essence, the plan contained in the bill we enacted last spring has four important parts.

First, there's malpractice insurance reform and malpractice liability reform. We attached it to the state plan for universal access so that it was all or nothing. It was hard to keep it in the bill. Opposition came from trial lawyers, low-income advocates, and the like. It starts with arbitration and then you can go to court if you want to, but the verdict from the arbitration proceeding is admissible as evidence in court and this dampens the willingness of a losing party to take a case to court. I do not expect malpractice insurance fees to drop; they're not high in the first place here. They're high for people in neurosurgery, orthopedics, and ob/gyn, but for the rest of us they are reasonable. Mine is about $2700 a year—not bad for an internist.

My real goal is to change the way we pay doctors in this state. I don't want us to reward doctors for doing more procedures, I want us to reward doctors for doing fewer procedures, or at least see to it that no additional income goes to anybody—hospitals or physicians—for doing unnecessary procedures. That's where I think the real money is to be saved in American medicine. But if we do that, it doesn't seem fair to retain a system of liability in which we encourage defensive medicine while we're paying people not to practice it.

The second part of our plan is to eliminate experience rating in the state. There has been none for large groups; it was eliminated for small groups; and now there is none for individuals. It's come one, come all.

We're also going to look at the profits of the insurance companies and enforce mandated loss ratios. If a company wants to sell health insurance in Vermont, its loss ratios will have to be at least 70 percent of what it takes in. A company just left Vermont because we did this. They were in the business of "cherry picking," that is, taking only the healthy folks and shifting all of the others elsewhere, either into the uninsured pool or into some other plan. Their loss ratio was 50 percent; half of every premium dollar they collected was theirs to keep. We didn't think that was serious insurance business and we didn't want that kind of stuff here. Originally I thought we were going to get down to three or four companies, which is really what I wanted. Now it looks like more will stay, and that's fine. We'll work with that.

Under the next provision, we will create a pool made up of public employees that is designed to have their insurance coverage negotiated in one big block. Private companies can buy into that approach, so that will establish some experience for us to get things up and running and to develop a system for buying health insurance.

The last provision established a Health Care Authority, and we've already put it in place. They're going to design a single-payer system and a multipayer system, and we will take both to the legislature in 1994 so that they can choose and pass one or the other. The first and toughest part of implementing the new bill was finding the three people to serve as the Authority. The necessary skills had to be there, and so did the right chemistry between the individuals. The dean of the University of Vermont's business school will chair it. A legislator who heads the commerce committee, and who was also one of the crafters and authors of the bill that we got through this year, will be one member, and the other will be the commissioner of social welfare, a person who also suggested many of the ideas in the bill.

While we were setting up the Authority, we reorganized several independent health care boards under the Authority and took other essential administrative steps. We doubled the number of uninsured children who were eligible for state health care by raising the age of covered children from 7 to 18. In addition, much earlier than we expected, we kicked into gear a safety net for people who need coverage because their insurers pulled out of Vermont in opposition to the new state laws outlawing experience rating.

Next, studies must be done of single-payer systems and of regulated multipayer systems for universal access to health care, and then, in 1994, the legislature must decide which system Vermont will establish. Common claim forms must be developed, and data must be collected by the Authority staff on such matters as hospital and insurance practices, costs, budgets, and so on. That will provide material the Authority will need to set global state health care budgets. Finally, the insurance purchasing pool, which is under a section of government separate from the Authority, must be created.

Physician incomes are not going to be capped, but we will have global budgeting. That means that the state will set a fixed amount of money that we will spend on health care for everybody in Vermont each year. After we do that, there will still be a two-tier health care system, and I really don't have a big problem with that. In all countries where there is universal access today, there is some sort of two-tier system. In Canada, which tries to legislate very hard against it, the two-tier system dictates that if you have the money, you can cross the border and get your care in the United States.

I don't think it's worth our time to worry about the 5 percent of the people who can take advantage of a two-tier system when we should be worrying about the 95 percent of the people who are either paying too much for health care or are unable to get any care at all. So I'm not going to get all hot and bothered about a two-tier system.

Under a state-sponsored insurance program, we would pay a certain amount. If a patient chose to pay more, fine. I'm not interested in controlling what physicians earn because that's not the troublesome issue. Sure, some doctors earn outrageous, ridiculous amounts of money and drive ostentatious cars, and I think those people would be better off working with mergers and acquisitions. But most physicians in Vermont, which ranks about 48th in the country in terms of what doctors earn, aren't in medicine for the money, and their income is not what's causing the problems; it's the procedures they order. If you come to my office for a $32 visit and leave with slips in your hand for $1600 worth of tests, it clearly is not my office visit that's running up the cost of health care. In some instances the doctor believes that the tests might help the patient, but too many of the tests are only marginally helpful.

It is the physician who should decide as to which tests are worthwhile and which are wasteful. The way I want this system to work is that you can come to my office and pay $32 if you want to see me, but I am going to have a specialist allowance. That is, if I order more tests and consultations than are covered by my global allowance for the year, then to learn why that happened I will be micromanaged during the next year by a utilization review board or some other bureaucratic organization. I think that micromanagement is awful, but I also think that a doctor who is threatened with having every chart gone over by a bureaucrat for a year will be a lot more careful about how much money he or she spends on tests. The other way to do this is through capitation. That is, we'll pay you so many dollars, and if you want to do 75 tests, be our guest. You will get the same amount of money whether you do one test or 75.

It is true that this sort of approach works against innovation in medicine and against the introduction of costly new modalities, and for a time Vermont will take advantage of technologies that are being developed elsewhere, just as other countries now take advantage of technologies that are being developed in the United States. Ultimately, when the whole country goes to universal health insurance, which it will be the end of this decade, we will have to have line items in the budget to provide for R&D. In fact, if the system works right in Vermont, eventually we will have line items in the budget for medical education and, perhaps, for R&D simply because now patient care dollars subsidize those activities—and that's not proper.

What we are doing in Vermont is definitely a model for the rest of the country. New York has already imitated our community rating system and passed an insurance bill modeled after ours. As for the continued growth of the science of medicine, if the federal government does what it should, if we have someone like Jimmy Carter in charge who is interested in funding the National Institutes of Health and the National Cancer Institute at the levels they should be funded, then research will continue to grow and prosper. But if we have an ignoramus in the White House, then little or nothing will be done about the future evolution of health care.

As we move ahead, difficult, value-based decisions will have to be made: if only once in, say, 10,000 studies of severe headache does an MRI scan detect a brain tumor early enough to save a life, is it worth the cost? I prefer to have those discussions take place at the level of the physician, the patient, and the family. We're going to pay physicians differently in Vermont so they're not going to be doing 10,000 MRI studies to find one brain tumor, but I wouldn't go so far as to adopt the Oregon system. There is a lot to be learned from it, but I don't think the government should decide what kind of health care we do and don't pay for. We ought to put significant budgetary constraints on physicians, patients, and families and then let them make the decisions in the contexts of those constraints.

Also, there's the problem of health care costs produced by large and intractable social problems, such as the costs of caring for sick babies born prematurely to teenage mothers who drink or take drugs. I don't know whether you can solve it or not. Our biggest cost problem in this country is that we're spending our money in the wrong places. The insurance structure currently pays for all the incredibly high-tech institutional care but not for mammograms, pap smears, or well-child visits. Nor does it pay very well for out-patient mental health care of home health care.

We'll spend $100,000 to transplant a baboon liver into one patient but we won't give any prenatal care to 100 women who are in the low-income category but are not qualified for Medicaid. That's crazy. We're spending our money totally backward. What we need to do is redesign the way we pay for medicine so that the system encourages all the preventive measures at the expense of the very high-tech stuff.

Now, what do you do about teenage pregnancy? We can't fix it with one magic step. This gets into other matters that we need to address, matters that I'm trying to deal with here in Vermont despite a horrendous budget problem. We need to get to kids at an early age. I want to integrate health care with educational and human services by having one-stop shopping. When you go to the doctor for postnatal care, the welfare, food stamp, alcohol and drug abuse, and family planning facilities will all be right there. So if you need them, you can get to them easily. Those are the kinds of things we need to be talking about, especially education.

As long as I'm governor, any health care proposal is going to be funded, at least in part, by tobacco and alcohol taxes. Why? Because people who use and abuse them clearly have higher health care bills, at least in the short term. That's yet to come, but it's part of our plan. Ironically, some studies show that tobacco smokers use less in the way of health care resources and die at a significantly earlier age. We have to do things with tax and fiscal policy, and with insurance program design, to get people to behave differently. By and large you accomplish that not by legislating it but by changing the economic rules to reward different behaviors in different ways.

It bothers many of us that eventually we may end up in this country refusing to pay for someone to get medical care of one type or another. There's always one more thing society can do. But we have finite resources, and the reason health care now consumes about 12 percent of the gross national product (and it's probably going to hit 20 percent in the next decade if we don't do something) is simply that we haven't faced up to making those choices. We're now trying to make those decisions here in Vermont. The budget level has to be set by society as a whole, and that is a political process. Then the individual choices have to be made within that context by the doctor and the patient.

The biggest problem is that the same person who wants to decree that we can no longer afford this or that treatment or test wants it all done, regardless of cost, when the illness involves himself or his family. Every time I talk about health care I talk about rationing. There's rationing now in every health care system in the world, including ours. We do it by price, but before too long there's going to be formal rationing. Americans have to get used to the idea that they can't have everything they want if they expect to control costs. It's something that the politicians have been terrified of telling the American people for a long time, but I think the American people are willing and ready to hear the truth.

If it's my personal problem, and I want a heart transplant but can't get it, and if we've got a democratic system in which I can get more than 50 percent of the people to agree that someone with my kind of medical problem should get a transplant, then we're going to have to spend more money on health care. If a majority won't vote to spend more money that way, then society won't pay for my transplant. If you have finite resources, you may have to make a choice between paying for a new liver for an 8-year-old child or paying for 100 women to get prenatal care. It's a tough choice, but it's got to be made.

A question underlying this choice is whether people want to spend money on such things as sports, entertainment, recreation, and the like, or whether they want to pay for health insurance. We're not going to give them the option. They're going to have to pay for health insurance under most systems because I think most people agree that if everybody is not insured, you don't have an insurance system that's going to work over the long term.

In a democracy such as ours, the people will have to make their own choice, and I think they will opt for health insurance for everyone. That will require a level of tax increases, and the people will have to define the level of tax increases with which they will be comfortable. That's what a democracy does. It works in a stumble-bum way, but at least it's a system in which everybody gets a say. Then if you vote for higher taxes to pay for health care, maybe you'll have less to spend on sports tickets. If you want low taxes, then you're going to get a low-cost medical system and all that it implies. People make such choices now when they decide whether to fund their schools or have sports people making millions of dollars a year.

One of the essential parts of my proposal is that the health care system will be administered by the state's government, but not, for God's sake, by the federal government. We already have a national health system in this country—Medicare—and it's a wonderful advertisement for why the federal government should never be allowed to run a national health care system. It's incredibly bureaucratic and mostly incompetent; the costs are completely out of control; and it's tremendously frustrating for patients and providers. It's a good model for what never to use.

In contrast, in small states you *can* use the Medicaid example. Medicaid is paid partly by the federal government. They set a broad band of guidelines that states can fit into, going either higher or lower, depending on their wishes. The state pays a proportion of it, and administers it, or, as with us, contracts with a private company to administer it, which works very well.

Doctors are unhappy about the reimbursement levels, and that has to be fixed. But doctors from the small states would be pleased to have universal health care run by the states or possibly contracted out. Doctors from large states have no more faith in state bureaucracy than they do in Washington, and I don't have a quick answer for them, unless you want to divide their states into multiple smaller administrative regions.

The only thing I didn't get legislated that I really wanted is approval for private employees to join the state's insurance pool right away. I felt it was essential to have full participation of the private sector, and I wanted the pool to be broad enough to include not just the purchasing pool but a risk pool as well. With that, we could set ourselves up in the insurance business and then contract out. I do not want this to be on the budget of the state. This is not going into a general fund to compete with roads and education.

I want health insurance in a separate, self-carrying fund, and I would like to contract it out to the private sector rather than have the state run it. If I could get away with it—and this is possible with a state our size—I would like to have the option of buying a policy from some company and having the company assume the risks and make any profits. Then we would be out of the insurance business. It's not my objective to get the state into the insurance business; my only objective is to make health insurance work for everybody.

Massachusetts had a plan for widening access to health insurance coverage, but when they started to implement it, they stopped. It was extraordinarily bureaucratic, poorly thought out, and done over the objections of the medical and hospital provider community. What we did here was to move a broad plan through with support from Democrats and Republicans. We could do that partly because everybody knows everybody in this state. Even though each person sticks up for his or her own business interests, there is a level of trust that doesn't exist in some larger states. There was also a radical movement toward immediate implementation of a single-payer system here, and that scared the pants off a lot of people and make our coalition much stronger. Our coalition represents about four-fifths of Vermont's population, and it's a broad consensus—Republicans, Democrats, large insurance companies, industry, providers, and many others.

I think, too, that it helped to have a governor who knew what he wanted and who knew how the political process works; this is my tenth year in public service. Having the medical degree certainly helped because I knew what I was talking about and had firm ideas about where I wanted to go. For example, I did not want a system of micromanagement because it reminds me too much of Medicare, is totally inefficient, and turns off providers. I hope to offer providers greater job satisfaction and less bureaucracy; I hope to offer business a substantial slowing of the increase in health care costs; and I hope to offer Vermont consumers the universal access that will remove their incredible feelings of insecurity about their ability to get adequate health care.

Universal access may require more money, but it may not. It certainly will not cost a staggering amount more because in Vermont everybody receives care now. Essentially, we have universal access; nobody gets turned away from hospitals and doctors. Occasionally it may happen in doctors' offices, but I don't believe it happens in any of Vermont's hospitals. The costs are simply passed on to the private sector through insurance payments. So, since everybody in Vermont receives health care, we don't have a huge amount of pent-up demand. Nevertheless there is some because Vermont is self-rationed in that Vermonters do not like to incur debt when they know they don't have the money to pay for it. Even though they know they would get the care anyway, they don't seek it. I hope that by using deductibles, copayments, and other things of that nature, we will be able to cope with the pent-up demand and have it canceled out by some real savings.

We need to get something into place in the legislature first and then see where the remaining problems are. Health care is a highly personal item for people, even more personal than land use planning or taxation, and people will pay attention. If they get upset, they'll speak up about it. There's no guarantee that it's all going to pass, but we're certainly as far along as anybody else, with the exception of Hawaii.

I have given up my medical practice for a while and I am running for governor, but at some point I would like to start taking care of patients again, at least part time. I could go back to practice, but I could also be in health care planning and health care policy somewhere. You make those other decisions when their time comes. I could have run for Congress in 1986 but I decided not to, partly because I certainly would have lost, but partly because I didn't want to move my family to Washington. We have young kids and Vermont is a wonderful place to grow up. We climb mountains and ski, which I make time for, especially now that the kids are a little older. At this point, I don't think it would be in the best interest of my family for us to move to Washington. Those considerations make a big difference when you're trying to think about where you're going. Besides, right now I've got a lot of work to do in this position.

I do not feel that I wasted my medical training by entering politics. If we manage to get universal care through here, I think I will have affected the health of far more people than I could have by working on a daily basis in the office. Medical education is all about accomplishing things for other people and helping them. There are ways to help people as a doctor other than by seeing them in the office.

I was always interested in politics, but if you had told me at the start that I would become governor of Vermont one day, I would have said that you were nuts. I don't have much time for myself these days. What I read is health economics, health politics, and budget documents. I do run and get exercise. I take time off for the kids, but I don't spend much time in solitude.

Chapter 25

SURGEON GENERAL

Dr. Joycelyn Elders was recruited by Governor Bill Clinton from her career as an academic pediatric endocrinologist to become director of the Arkansas Health Department and then by President Clinton to become the surgeon general of the U.S. Public Health Service, a position she left in December 1994. The interview for this chapter was done just as she was getting ready to leave Arkansas for Washington. The subsequent course of events has received enough attention in the media to warrant no further comment here.

Joycelyn Elders, M.D., Pediatrician in an academic medical center, Health Care Administration

I tried to do especially well in school so I could get out of the cotton patch. . . . I was having a good time in pediatric endocrinology and . . . then Governor Clinton asked me to be director of health for Arkansas. . . . What I have pushed the most on are early childhood education, comprehensive health education for K through 12, parenting education, teaching young men to be responsible fathers, making services available in school where the children are . . . and giving hope.

The oldest of eight children, I grew up on an Arkansas farm where we raised the three "C's": cotton, corn, and cattle. Because I had to help with the field work, I tried to do especially well in school so I could get out of the cotton patch. It was a difficult challenge for any of us to make it to college. I received a scholarship to Philander Smith College, a school in Little Rock supported by the United Methodist Church. I was able to go to college only because, as class valedictorian, I got help with tuition and part of my room and board costs. Even so, my sisters and brothers had to pick extra cotton so I could pay for the bus fare to Little Rock and start school. I made a commitment to myself that if any of them wanted to go to college, they would do so just as long as I could help. Six of them went. They never minded working; I had to work hard too, but they went to state-supported schools, got tuition paid, bought used books, and worked for room and board. This experience led me eventually to urge Arkansas's governor to pay for tuition and books for our bright young people without scholarships. The legislature passed it and even put money into it, an important investment in the future of our state.

My high school was a country school, and most students took every course. Our school did its best to offer the basics. All of our teachers were black. Back then, and even now, advisors counseled students not to consider a career in medicine because we weren't good enough. We didn't have radio or television to open our horizons, and when I left home my highest aspiration was to become a lab technician. I got that idea during World War II when my parents went to California to work in the Henry Kaiser shipyards. There in junior high school I saw people working in a lab and felt that being a lab technician was absolutely at the top of the stars.

Then, when I was a college freshman, a young woman came to talk to us. She was a sophomore in medical school—the first black woman to attend the University of Arkansas—and she talked about the difference between the high road and the low road. I decided to be just like her and become a doctor.

My college, a United Methodist school for black students, consisted of a faculty who, though not inclined to discourage us, were realists. They did not think our chances of doing something like attending medical school were the greatest in the world, so they tried to make sure that we took enough education courses to become teachers. They thought that was the safe direction for us.

I finished college in 3 years, but my parents could not afford to send me to medical school so I didn't even consider it a possibility. Since I was pretty smart then (not like now), I decided to go into the service and use the GI bill to go to medical school. In the service, I trained as a physical therapist and was commissioned as a first lieutenant. I stayed in the army until I had accumulated enough time to cover medical school. The military experience helped me to mature and I enjoyed it. For the first time I was in a more integrated environment. There were 18 of us, all women college graduates, who went into physical therapy. I was the only black woman. These women were wonderful friends and eventually five of us went on to medical school.

When the time came to apply to medical school, I felt I had the best chance of getting into the University of Arkansas. However, I applied to the University of Colorado too and was accepted at both places. I chose Arkansas because it was home and because it was a little cheaper.

It wasn't easy then to be black and in medical school in Arkansas, but maybe our skins were very thick. I was in medical school during the uproar about Central High School and the school integration crisis. When we started out, we could not sit in the dining room with the other medical students. We had to eat in the dining room reserved for the cleaning staff. There were three blacks, two men and me, in a class of about 100. There were only three women in all. Both black men graduated with the class, but I was the only woman to do so. We women lived together. At one point some neighbors told one of the white women that she shouldn't live with me. My classmate said that she would be happy to move if they would pay her rent; we stayed together until she married and moved to St. Louis to become a radiologist.

At first I thought I wanted to be a family physician. However, in my senior year a young female pediatrician suggested that I enter pediatrics and train at the University of Minnesota, at that time considered one of the best pediatric internships in the country. She and her husband had interned there. Just before she came along, I had wanted to become a pediatric surgeon because I enjoyed surgery so much. The truth is, I enjoyed everything in medical school. I wanted to be an obstetrician, I wanted to be a pediatrician, and I wanted to be a surgeon, but I decided to be a pediatric surgeon because there weren't many around.

I got married during my senior year. My husband is a high school basketball coach from Arkansas. When I was a senior, I went over to examine his basketball team and I've been examining his teams ever since. I was so flattered to be accepted for the internship at the University of Minnesota that even though we were married, I went to Minnesota and spent the year there. It was painful to come back because Minnesota had a pediatric surgery residency program. But it was more difficult to be away from my husband, so I gave up surgery, came home, and enjoyed pediatrics. If we had settled in Minnesota, I would have become a pediatric surgeon, like Koop.

I was considering becoming a practitioner, but when I was chief resident a faculty member who was in research recommended that I do a fellowship. So I started working in his lab. He was a wonderful mentor. I happened to be in the right place at the right time, and I got pregnant at the right time too. My mentor was in pathology and I did a rotation with him. He kept saying, "What are you going to do next? You don't want to go out and practice. You need to be a teacher." He pushed and pulled, and finally I decided to do the fellowship. After I got my fellowship award, he insisted that I go back and learn some chemistry. "You don't know anything," he told me. I went back and nearly completed a PhD in biochemistry. I got a masters degree in biochemistry at Arkansas during my 3-year postdoctoral fellowship, and I had a child in the third year.

The year I was chief resident, I was at the hospital 7 days a week. I never missed a day, but I enjoyed it and didn't think it was bad at the time. A wonderful lady with whom we stayed for 4 months when we first got married came to feel that she was our mother. After the baby came, she took care of us for years. When I had to go to work nights, she kept the baby, which was terrific. I didn't realize I had such a good thing until later on.

Then I got a 5-year NIH Career Development Award in endocrinology, my mentor's field. He told me that as a resident I had spent 4 years taking care of patients and that in my fellowship my only job was to do research and to learn something about chemistry and statistics. He was pointing me in the direction of academic medicine, which was kind of appealing. I enjoyed teaching and taking care of patients. When I started in research, I had to take biochemistry with freshman medical students. After having been chief resident it was hard to be in a beginner's course.

When I became an endocrinologist, I was the first board-certified pediatric endocrinologist in Arkansas. I became the director of the endocrinology training program and had to take care of a lot of children with diabetes. My major research was related to growth problems, which I worked on for 20 years. I became a full professor in 1976, probably the first black professor and the first black female professor. By then the school took pride in having a black female on their faculty; they would trot me out for recruitment purposes.

We never had more than five to seven black students per class of 100. There weren't many young black college students who felt they could get into medical school or succeed there. Then the school hired a dean of minority students to try to increase minority enrollment, which is now up to 10–15 percent. The population of minorities in Arkansas is about 12 percent.

I was having a good time in pediatric endocrinology. I'd done all the things that medical academics do, and I was settled and very happy. Then Governor Bill Clinton asked me to be director of health for Arkansas. When President Clinton was the state's attorney general, my best friend, a lawyer, introduced my husband and me to the Clintons. Later on, Mrs. Clinton served on commissions and boards to which the governor appointed me, and whenever he wanted me to do something I didn't want to do, he would have her call me. She would say, "Joycelyn, Bill really wants you to do this and it is the most important commission of his administration (everything was 'the most important' to him) and we really need you to do this." That's one of her roles, and she does it as well as he does.

She was interested in children's issues from the very beginning. Although her major focus was education, she was quite interested in health because she knew that you can't educate children if they aren't healthy and you can't keep them healthy if they aren't educated. She has a sincere and deep commitment to improving the health and education of children.

When President Clinton was governor and asked me to be the director of the Health Department for the state, it was something I had never planned to do. I told him that I would only consider it if I could retain my tenured professorship at the university, if I got a 10 percent salary increase, and if he would really let me run the department. I was being facetious. I didn't think he would do any of it. But 3 weeks later he called in the middle of the night and said, "Joycelyn, I've got it all done. Will you take it?" I answered, "Oh my, I said I would, didn't I?" He said, "Yes, you did!" I said, "Well, I guess I'm not going to become a liar." He said, "Thanks! Bye."

I had never had any intention of doing it, but I started in October of 1987, and these have been the most wonderful 5 years I've ever spent. I have been able to make policy, to increase public awareness, to force change, to hire people to work with me who are ready and willing to change things, and to make things happen for children in this state. I think I've probably done more for children in the past 5 years than I ever did during the previous 20.

I direct a centralized health department, but I am also responsible for public health workers throughout the state and must cover such areas as water quality, our huge in-home health service, and environmental issues related to public health. When I came I had to learn about plumbing, health care facilities, hospitals, and other subjects about which I didn't know much.

My most important goal, to reduce teenage pregnancy in Arkansas, was our most difficult challenge. We're getting a program in place, and in addition I got the fundamentalist religious right groups to understand that we need to do things that will make a difference. We have to start with early childhood education so that young people will do well in school, feel good about themselves, and look forward to the future. I obtained funding to begin to do some of those things.

I started out by pushing at the social and economic levels. I felt that we had to do six things; if we did only five it would be like having a leaky bucket with five holes plugged and the sixth one unplugged: we'd still have a leaky bucket. What I have pushed the most on are early childhood education, comprehensive health education from K through 12, parenting education, teaching young men to be responsible fathers by, for example, getting them to enter their social security numbers in the records along with their children's birth certificates so we can always know where to find them, making services available in school where the children are (we've built many school-based clinics), and giving hope. We got legislation passed to provide tuition and books for young people with a B average or above who want to go to college and who come for families with incomes of $25,000 or less. It's taken me all 5 years to get these moving, and though I don't have them fully funded, we've received money for all of them. It will take more time, however, because we need to change the basic fabric of our state.

Both Clintons have been supportive. When I'd been health director for just 3 weeks, he and I held a press conference together and I was asked what the Health Department was going to do to help adolescents. I said that we were going to reduce teenage pregnancy by having health education and school-based clinics. Then the press asked me whether we were going to provide condoms at schools, and I said, "We're not going to put them on the lunch trays, but, yes." The governor turned red. His mouth fell open, and he just sat there. The press turned away from me and said, "Governor, Dr. Elders just said. . . . " and they repeated my answer. He sat there for a minute, swallowed a few times, and replied, "Dr. Elders told me what she was about when I appointed her, and I want you to know that I support Dr. Elders." That took courage, and you know he never changed.

He never said anything to me about my approach, but I'm sure he was taken aback at first. Still, he fought for it and did the best he could to help. Just recently, he said, "Well, Dr. Elders, I know you didn't get everything you wanted for Arkansas, but I think it will all happen. It will just take longer than you thought." But, directly out of general revenues, he put $10 million into early childhood education, he put $5 million a year into support for college education, and he put money into school-based clinics.

The challenges are problems of poverty, but they seem worse because the poverty is higher among blacks than whites in our society. Homelessness, drug addiction, and the like are part and parcel of the same thing. If we start early with the children, make them feel good about themselves and with school, if schools are committed and are providing the necessary services, then we'll have a better chance of preventing problems. We would be far better off funding prevention than we are now chasing after the problems and trying to fix them.

I told my brother, a United Methodist minister, that the churches needed to stop moralizing from the pulpit and preaching to the choir. They need to go into the street and get to work. It took a while but they became committed, which has been a great help. One minister became chairman of the minority AIDS commission; some joined the task force on teen pregnancy; and at their annual conference the United Methodist Churches of Arkansas adopted resolutions to work on the problems of teen pregnancy and youth suicide. In addition, a media campaign called "Hold Out the Lifeline" was presented in local churches to try to reduce infant mortality.

Then I had to reach the schools. The schools were worse than the streets. They felt that their job was to teach reading, writing, and arithmetic and that they had no other responsibilities. Schools have social, moral, and educational responsibilities, but they can't teach young people who aren't physically, emotionally, and psychologically ready to learn. Because children are in school all day, the schools of the 21st century must be a place where they can have all of their social, emotional, and educational needs met. The school is where we interact with the parents. It's the only place where all of the children have to go. If we don't address the problems, we're going to have wonderful things for the children of parents who probably don't need that much help, whereas the children who need it the most will always be left behind.

If I move to Washington, most of these ideas will be transferable. We hope to fund early childhood education nationally and deal with Head Start. The President feels strongly about early childhood education and will treat it as a priority. There will be a big push for a merger of health and education, which is already happening in Washington. I was on the secretary's committee to look at health and education under President Bush's administration. We had only two meetings, but the idea is to put through a comprehensive health education program. We can accomplish 30 percent of the national health objectives by the year 2000 by working with primary and secondary schools.

Some of the problems in Arkansas are as bad as those in sections of Brooklyn or downtown Los Angeles; they're just not as concentrated. I wish I knew how to reach the inner cities. I've been impressed with how well we do when we draw the community into schools to try to solve kids' problems. They come to view the schools as their own. They need to feel that this is "my nurse," "my clinic," "my social worker," and "my psychiatrist," and that they can drop by those facilities even without any money. These approaches work and are far cheaper than the benign neglect we've had thus far.

Whatever happens in the future, it's still going to be fun to be a doctor. We have a real lack of primary care physicians. We have focused too much of our funds and efforts on the last few months of life rather than on preventive services and the many other areas where we can make a lasting difference. We have to change our focus.

We won't have enough generalists until we look at how we pay them. Right now, a doctor can get up at 3 A.M. to see somebody with pneumonia, take an X-ray, start treatment, comfort the family, stay up all night, and get paid far less than the radiologist who gets up the next morning and reads the film in 5 minutes. If that keeps up, we won't have many young doctors going into primary care in rural areas where nobody has any money.

As already implied, we don't do enough preventive health care. We don't pay for counseling teenagers to prevent pregnancy but we pay readily for the care of a low-birth-weight baby. You can't get through to a teenager in a 5-minute conversation. No one will pay for the kind of time doctors need for counseling and talking to adolescents.

In some respects more attention must be paid to nurse practitioners. We have a lot of them in the Health Department here in Arkansas, and it works. Indeed, sometimes we doctors don't do as well as nurse practitioners when it comes to counseling and interacting with people. We know our medicine and can handle the technical aspects, but when we get to the humanistic aspects we have a lot to learn.

When I was taking care of children with diabetes, we had to reassure the mothers, teach them how to take care of their children, manage the diets, and do everything necessary to ensure that the children were receiving the proper care. Often, if a child was having trouble and I answered the phone, the parent would say, "Dr. Elders, I want to talk to Francine." She was my nurse practitioner. I would say, "Well, you can ask me, I have time right now." And the parent would respond, "That's all right, let me talk to Francine." My ego took a beating, but they knew that Francine would take care of them or come to me if she couldn't.

If I go to Washington, I will return to Arkansas when I'm finished there. I'm 59 and have promised myself retirement at 62. When I retire, I will go home and raise watermelons. We live on a 15-acre farm, about 15 minutes from my office. We love it and raise lots of vegetables there. We've lived in Arkansas all our lives and it's a good place to live. Everybody who comes here is always pleasantly surprised. Maybe it's because they expect that it will be so terrible. We have a disproportionate share of elderly people living in our state because so many move here. They've developed a community that caters to the upper middle class and middle income elderly. We like having them because they can pay for what they want.

Helping people to grow old with dignity, to receive decent health care, and to die somewhere other than in an intensive care unit is critical. Putting folks in nursing homes early is not an answer. Perhaps we can train younger people in the community, who, let's say, are on welfare, to provide services for elderly people in their own homes. In our Health Department we do a lot to support that kind of personal care.

When it comes to research, we should make funds available to the limits of our ability. I have concerns about such questions as whether we are pushing harder in AIDS research than we have knowledge or capability. We shouldn't overinvest in one area because we're desperate for an answer. Often the things we learn in one area help us to find answers in another. We shouldn't say that if anybody has an idea related to AIDS that they should test it; the scientists know whether it makes sense and is a good idea. We should consider it in that vein rather than simply allocating large funds for AIDS research.

AIDS treatment should be under health care reform, not the research budget. It looks as though all this money is being spent on research and public health when in fact it's being spent on treatment. So far as basic research goes, the one area where we're making a big mistake is in not training, developing, and providing more research opportunities for young people. If I were starting out today, I might not be given the opportunity that I had earlier. We're losing excellent young people because of a lack of funding and we aren't even training them in basic research. That's where we're losing out most heavily.

I'm not a person who believes in spending more money, more money, and more money; nevertheless, I'll have to become as good a lobbyist as those in the defense industry. That's a tall order because they've been at it a lot longer. We've got to have a strong defense capability, but when you look at the percentage of the defense budget that goes into research and development and the percentage of what we put into research and development from the medical end, there's no comparison.

In putting the house of medicine in order, let's start with premature babies. If we make a real investment so that every child born in America becomes a planned and wanted child, that will have an important impact. That's something we can't afford to neglect.

And then, at some point it becomes time to die. I don't know when that is—and I'm not trying to know—but too often we don't allow our elderly people to die with dignity and instead prolong their life when it's not even a life they would like. The quality of life on tubes and needles for months is not very attractive. I don't know when, where, and how to pull the plug, but we need to think about it. If a doctor were to start inserting tubes and needles in my mother-in-law, I think I'd sue. The best thing for her is to be kept comfortable and free of pain, and one day to go to sleep and not wake up.

I would like young people to feel that medicine is a wonderful profession, but we must never forget that we are taking care of people. We should not see dollar signs painted on our eyeballs before we learn about the human need for care and compassion.

Chapter 26

EDITOR OF A MAJOR MEDICAL JOURNAL

Few medical publications reach as many physician and even lay readers throughout the world as the *New England Journal of Medicine*. Its editor-in-chief enjoys an unparalleled opportunity to learn about new developments in biomedical science and technology, health care policy, and social issues; to create important settings for discussions of questions related to these subjects; and to enter into the various debates. It is most unlikely that when Dr. Relman began his clinical training in what later became the clinical discipline of nephrology he anticipated that his career would bring him to the editor's chair.

Dr. Arnold S. Relman is the editor-in-chief emeritus of the *New England Journal of Medicine* and professor emeritus of medicine and of social medicine at Harvard Medical School. He devotes most of his professional time to writing and public speaking.

Arnold S. Relman, M.D., Nephrologist, Academician, Editor

The current discomfort and unhappiness among physicians is a temporary inevitable manifestation of a major transition in the organization and orientation of medical care in this country. The role of the physician will not change, and the satisfactions that physicians get from the practice of medicine will always be there. In fact, medicine will grow even

more exciting as the power of physicians to diagnose, pre-
vent, and treat diseases increases. This is a wonderful time
to get into medicine, and I see no reason for despair.

I was born in New York City, went to public schools there, and got my undergraduate college degree from Cornell. Somewhere along the line, I read *Microbe Hunters* and *Arrowsmith* and entered college as a premedical student. I went to Columbia University College of Physicians and Surgeons and took my residency training at Yale.

After that, in 1949, I took a fellowship at Boston University in electrolyte physiology, salt and water metabolism, acid-base balance, and renal disease. "Nephrology" had not been invented yet. I wanted to do research, teach, and see patients. After a year, my chief left and, much to my surprise, I was asked to take over as head of endocrinology, nephrology, and metabolic diseases. One of my colleagues was Franz Ingelfinger.

I stayed there from 1949 to 1968 and edited the *Journal of Clinical Investigation* from 1962 to 1967. I became increasingly interested in medical editing and was appointed to the Committee on Publications of the *New England Journal of Medicine*. While I was serving on it, Joe Garland, the editor, retired and we selected Franz Ingelfinger to succeed him.

In 1968 I became chairman of medicine at the University of Pennsylvania where I stayed for 9 years. I kept in close touch with Franz Ingelfinger. He told me that he had the best job in American medicine but that 10 years would probably be enough. Sadly, in his tenth year, he had to resign for health reasons. I was on a sabbatical leave at Oxford at the time, and early in 1976 I was invited to take up Franz's post.

I accepted but with misgivings about being able to live up to the Garland and Ingelfinger traditions. I stayed for 14 years, until 1991, when I retired to write and teach at Harvard. The editorship afforded me an unmatched opportunity to observe American medicine and the health care system from the broadest possible perspective, away from intense involvement in my clinical field and my particular institution. The job gave me an opportunity to speak out on medical policy issues and to influence that debate. It also allowed me to keep up with the cutting edge of medicine.

Getting the journal out demanded constant attention. An enormous mass of material and information pours into the editor's office — phone messages, manuscripts, complex issues — and the editor needs to deal with people, personalities, reporters, institutions, politics, economics, ethics, law, and even commerce. It was all systole with no diastole, and I was glad I put it down when I did. I had withdrawal symptoms for a while, but now I have time to myself to think, work on issues, and write a book.

I have three children, a physician son in research and two lawyers, and five grandchildren. I would absolutely encourage any of my grandchildren to seek a career in medicine if that interests them. Medicine will always be a wonderful profession. The current discomfort and unhappiness among physicians is a temporary inevitable manifestation of a major transition in the organization and orientation of medical care in this country. The role of physician will not change, and the satisfactions that physicians get from the practice of medicine will always be there. In fact, medicine will grow even more exciting as the power of physicians to diagnose, prevent, and treat diseases increases. This is a wonderful time to get into medicine, and I see no reason for despair.

For several reasons, in the debate about health care policy the voices of medicine are not being listened to sufficiently. Economists, political scientists, and politicians have captured the field because the urgent need to control costs and to extend health care to everyone seems to call for political and economic solutions. Also, there is an unfortunate and widespread perception that doctors have acted too much as a special interest group. Yes, we have championed universal access and improved quality, but until recently we haven't addressed today's overriding issue, cost control; so we've not been invited to the table. We should be because without physician participation and cooperation one can't have a health care system.

I hope that the process will play out rationally, but it's too early to tell. What will happen after a plan for health care reform is put forward is anybody's guess. Closely related to the central issue of controlling costs is the problem of the 38 million Americans without health insurance. Most of them get some kind of health care but it isn't very good. In many ways the insurance that the rest of us have is also inadequate — not comprehensive or stable enough, and too restrictive in that it usually fails to cover the full range of risks that we all face, including catastrophic or prolonged illness. If we could control costs, we could probably afford to insure everybody.

Another problem is the terrible inefficiency of the system. It is wasteful, duplicative, and undermined by fraud and profiteering. We spend more than any other country by far but get a product that is not uniformly satisfactory—even though at its best, American health care is unsurpassed in the world.

There's no simple answer, and there may not even be a not-so-simple answer. The roots of the problem penetrate the entire structure of the American society and economy, and involve the conflicting interests of many powerful elements. Instead of a system with a uniform, organizing principle that can be dealt with as a whole, we have a nonsystem, a helter-skelter hodgepodge of ad hoc arrangements that offer differential benefits, profits, and advantages to a vast number of interested parties.

Many call it an industry now, and if it is one, it's the largest in the country, consuming better than 14 percent of the economy and growing at about 10 percent per year. In this year alone, the cost of health care will rise by over $100 billion. Because the system employs more than 10 million people and supports many thousands of businesses, the magnitude of divergent interests makes it impossible to get a single hold on the problem or find one lever that will move the system.

Different analysts have different ideas about what is causing the runaway cost inflation in health care, but here are some of the major factors. Until now we have had a largely cost or charge reimbursement system that is paid for by third parties. The benefits go to the patient, who generally pays only 20 percent out of the pocket and so the usual elements of consumer restraint and choice are absent. Not only do the third parties pay on a piece-work reimbursement basis, but the number and nature of the covered items are determined not by the consumer or the third-party payer but by the physician, the very one who stands to benefit substantially from the number and type of services being provided. This peculiar system is an open invitation to inflation.

There's more. The products being sold and provided are becoming much more numerous, sophisticated, and expensive. The new techniques, test, procedures, and drugs usually come out of investor-owned corporations with a major stake in marketing their products. In addition, doctors are growing more numerous in relation to the population, and the kinds of doctors we produce now are about 80 percent specialists trained to use specialized tests and procedures; their professional careers depend on the new technology for which somebody else is paying. On top of that, the medical indications for the clinical value and use of the particular services, drugs, operations, and tests are inadequately understood and tested. Clinical investigation and technology assessment are going on but at a rate far below that at which the new modalities are being advanced.

Although physicians get paid only 20 cents of the health care dollar, their decisions and recommendations determine the expenditure of at least 75 to 80 percent of the rest of the dollar, and their decisions are made without clear-cut information about what is worth the money and which approach is more effective. The imperative to do whatever might possibly help is reinforced by an economic inducement to do it and by the knowledge that the patient usually doesn't have to pay very much. Given all of these factors, it amazes me that health care costs are going up only at the rate of $100 billion a year.

Aging of the population is a factor but not a big one. On average, people over 65 use about two and one half times as much health care resources as people under 65. At present, about 12 percent of the population is over 65. In 30 years it will be 15–18 percent. By simple arithmetic, it's a small factor.

Social pathology is a major factor, but it's hard to put a number on it. Without question, an enormous amount of money is spent trying to contain the medical damage we do to ourselves through alcoholism, smoking, drug abuse, violence by guns, highway accidents, and so on. Poverty, ignorance, lack of education, and disruption of American family life contribute greatly. That is why although we think that our medical care capacity is increasing all the time, and we spend more money on medical care, the health outcomes, as measured by such public health parameters as longevity, length of life, infant mortality, or percentage of kids being vaccinated, don't measure up very well.

Many of our problems are largely social, political, and economic in origin, and the doctors are left to deal with the consequences. But medical care, as opposed to public health programs, is designed primarily to deal with acute conditions, to prevent death or disability from urgent problems, to comfort even when a cure isn't possible, to diagnose and sort out difficulties, and simply to add to the quality of life. If you're really interested in preserving as many infants as possible, you will do something about teenage pregnancy, poverty in inner cities and rural areas, drug abuse, and so forth.

Like many other people, I have a fairly clear notion of an ideal system. The question is how to get from where we are today to where we'd like to be. No single law that Congress is likely to pass in the foreseeable future and no single stroke of the president's pen is going to solve the problem.

The system I would like to see in place by the end of the decade would look something like this: everyone, regardless of age, sex, employment status, disability status, medical condition, or what not, would be covered by a universal insurance system that would provide a defined, reasonable package of comprehensive health care benefits. The package might have to be modified as we develop more experience, but it would certainly include most of the essential elements of health or medical care.

The money would come from a national medical fund, which, like the social security fund, would be kept discrete from other national funds. Everyone would contribute to it according to their means through an identifiable surtax on income tax or through a payroll tax. The money would be earmarked only for expenses directly related to medical care, such as the cost of prepaid medical coverage provided by a private sector HMO system, and the cost of backing up the prepayment system through a reinsurance mechanism for protecting HMOs against adverse risk and unusual catastrophic illness.

Every organized health care plan or HMO would be required by law to accept anyone as a member regardless of whether the person has AIDS, advanced liver disease, chronic alcoholism, whatever. HMOs would be paid a premium based on a national allocation established as reasonable for covering the average costs of comprehensive care. The premium would be adjusted for variations in local cost of living, segment of the population covered, and patient mix. There would also have to be a provision for catastrophes.

These health care plans would be not-for-profit, community-centered cooperatives, owned not by insurance companies, for-profit businesses, or doctors working in them but by the consumers who would have voting rights and be represented by a board of directors of the HMO. A fraction of the total amount of money collected by the HMO (based perhaps on what doctors earn now, namely, on average 11 percent after expenses) would be set aside for doctors, who would determine their salaries from that fixed pool.

HMOs would be required by law to hire a specified number of

staff doctors per member, a number derived from present experience with well-run HMOs. In addition to salaries, the doctors would receive appropriate fringe benefits, including malpractice insurance coverage, retirement benefits, educational expenses, office expenses, and so on.

From the start, the consumer owners of the HMO would put the 11 percent on the table and tell the doctors, "That's your money to manage. You set your salaries and administer the fund. For that money, it will be your responsibility, not Uncle Sam's or an insurance company's, to manage our medical care. You are to keep us healthy, provide the medical care that you think is justified, and be accountable for it."

There would also be regional and possibly national purchasing cooperatives for supplies, equipment, and pharmaceuticals. Each region would have a quasi-public independent agency like the Federal Reserve Broad to watch over the HMOs by setting standards for accountability and record keeping, by making sure that there were no abuses, and by arbitrating and mediating disputes and problems. Its first responsibility would be to certify the HMOs in the region that meet requirements. If an HMO ran in the red, the board would evaluate whether the deficit was justified because of medical or social factors, or whether it was attributable to mismanagement.

My plan does not involve price competition; that tends to undermine standards of quality and to create an instability that is not conducive to sustaining community service and doctor–patient relations. In many not-for-profit health care institutions price competition and hard Darwinian rivalry have bred unhealthy entrepreneurial attitudes. The patient does not know how to make wise choices in a health care setting based on such competition. That's why there would be no price competition, and prices would be fixed by a national health board with representation from consumers and providers. It would estimate reasonable average per capita health care costs and might define the appropriate range of services by learning what HMOs all over the country have been able to do.

The Board would say something like this to the doctors: "We will pay you $2500 per capita per year (a big savings over what is spent today), modified according to local conditions. If you can live within that budget and provide satisfactory service as advocates for your patients and as discriminating and compassionate dispensers of medical services, you will be rewarded in the way that health care providers traditionally have been rewarded—by the confidence and trust of your patients, and you will have as many patients as you want." If money is left over at the end of the year, the HMO might use it to improve facilities and services. There would be no bonuses or other monetary rewards beyond salaries but salaries should reflect the quality of each physician's contribution to the group effort. If an HMO finished in the red, the regional Board would examine the cause. They would explore whether the correction for patient mix and severity of illness was inadequate. If so, they would increase the payment to the HMO. If the HMO's administrative overhead was out of line or a lot of money was wasted, they would work with the HMO to improve its operations and keep it in business.

Medical care will be managed by doctors, although technically the HMO will be owned by the consumers. When there isn't money to cover a procedure, a doctor will use his or her best judgment. If most HMOs in a region finished in the red, more tax revenues would be needed. Then it would come down to a simple choice: either the public would agree to pay more for the services, or they would decide they cannot afford to pay for, let's say, all the MRIs the doctors want. There will be no free lunch, no way to provide services without somebody paying for it.

Healthy consumers may see no need to insure themselves, but when they become sick, they may demand more tests and all forms of treatment, regardless of cost. They may be unwilling to pay for a health insurance plan that covers everyone, rich or poor, sick or well. The question is whether we are willing to live in a society where the healthy allow the sick poor to suffer. Without a collective sense of responsibility we cannot have an equitable health care system except under a bureaucratic, government-dictated system. I don't want that and neither do most people. I may be unrealistic and idealistic, but I believe in the common sense and decency of the American people. Once the facts are clear and people see that nobody is trying to gain any advantage over anybody else, and that everybody is in the same boat, they may do the right thing. I believe they will see the need for us all to share the financial responsibility for universal health insurance, according to our ability to pay.

The medical care fund must also cover the costs of technology assessment, outcome evaluation, medical education and training, and clinical research. These are so closely related to the quality of clinical health services as to constitute a legitimate R&D expense for this vast industry. The medical care fund will be so huge that these added costs will be a drop in the bucket. A highly technological industry like health care can certainly afford to allocate 10 percent of its gross annual expenditures (about $90 billion) for these purposes. Basic biomedical research, which is mainly the NIH's responsibility, ought to be funded separately.

Technology assessment is a national responsibility. For FDA approval, I would require not only that drugs and devices be tested for safety and effectiveness but that they be assessed in comparison with existing technology or drugs. I am opposed not only to government takeover of the delivery of medical services but to the takeover of the manufacture of drugs and medical equipment. As an essential part of the delivery system, the drug companies should remain privately owned. They should make a fair profit and have enough money to support R&D but not enough to support today's level of marketing and promotion. Since drugs for the HMOs will be purchased wholesale with critical assessment of what is worth the money, marketing programs aimed mainly at individual physicians will become less important. Sales will be sustained only if the drugs are good and useful products. Smaller firms may go out of business, but the major players with sound basic research will continue to do well. To avoid excessive price increases or windfall profits, the government could regulate the annual rate of pharmaceutical price inflation by holding it to something like no more than 1 percent over the rise in the cost of living.

I do not envision HMOs as the only approach to health care; I envision options. I described a system to which everybody would contribute through taxes, like public education, but there should be other choices for care. If you wanted to buy more insurance, such as total coverage with indemnification payments to physicians and hospitals of your own choosing, you should be free to do so. However, within the next 5 years the cost of full indemnification private coverage could well be over $25,000 a year for a family of four—out of range for all but a small minority of the population. Almost everyone will have to depend on prepaid HMO-type coverage for most or all of their health care.

Most Americans will stay with the basic coverage and most physicians will find their only practice opportunities within that system, which is strong protection against deterioration of the basic system and bureaucratic neglect. A system that is mainly for poor people will lack powerful advocates and defenders. Like Medicaid, it can become very shabby. A system involving most doctors and consumers, and supported by an earmarked tax that does not go into the general government revenues, will have a far better chance of maintaining good standards.

In addition to opting for complete separate coverage, people could supplement their coverage, as occurs with Medicare now. If you want access to specialists outside your HMO, you should have it, provided you pay an additional premium. Some people argue against allowing anybody to opt out, especially congresspersons and government workers, because you run the risk of having the rich and the powerful getting their care from another system and having no interest in protecting the quality of the basic one. That is a concern, but if most people are in the system there is a good possibility that they will keep it from deteriorating.

With this model there will be two kinds of hospitals. Most will be community hospitals, providing mainly secondary care and a little tertiary care, and doing little or no teaching or research. Wherever possible, the HMOs will own them. About 120,000 HMO members will keep a 150- to 175-bed community hospital comfortably filled. Because an HMO's premiums will cover hospital expenses, its doctors will be motivated to use hospital resources prudently. Hospitals that contract with HMOs will have to offer uniform per diem rates so that a hospital won't be able to play one HMO off against another.

The other kind of hospital will be the tertiary care, teaching, and research hospitals. They should be regional resources receiving their support from several different sources. They should be paid set fees for certain specialized services—so much for a heart transplant, for example. The fee negotiation would be conducted with the regional Health Board and individual HMOs needing to use those services would be indemnified by the Board for adverse selection and for unusual risk.

Another source of payment for the teaching hospital would be a fund for research and education maintained by the regional Board. There would be a budget for training house staff, nurses, technicians, and so on, and for technology assessment. To train medical students, a teaching hospital would want to have an HMO affiliated with it. The hospital would also need a staff of primary care practitioners large enough to run its clinics. I don't want to minimize the task; there will be difficult problems to solve. In principle, it should be possible to say to a teaching hospital, "We want you to teach medical students how to practice primary care and how to work in a group setting like an HMO since that is where most of them will practice afterward. Therefore, you need to maintain a teaching HMO, and that will be more expensive. Just as we correct for patient care mix and for adverse selection, so, too, will we need to adjust your budget for teaching costs."

Today's HMOs are a mixed bag. They have had different incentives; few are cooperatives. Most are for-profit investor-owned companies that contract with doctors and find it difficult to control costs. Many have been badly managed by heavy-handed business administrators who look primarily at the bottom line and who tell doctors how to care for their patients. The system I propose would include only not-for-profit HMOs with no incentives to underserve or overserve patients.

Past experience with HMOs has been spotty. Some have been outstandingly successful, as judged by cost control, quality, and acceptance by patients and doctors; some have been terrible to the point of running afoul of the law; and we've had everything in between. HMOs have lacked incentive to be as efficient as possible because with relatively little effort, simply by using hospitals less, they can offer lower premiums than indemnification insurers. HMOs are still in the minority, with only some 50 million people now enrolled, but membership is increasing rapidly. HMOs have to keep their premiums below those of their competition, but since HMO prices can follow the competition's rising prices, HMOs can easily accede to the demand for fancy technology and more use of services. The well-organized and well-managed HMOs are very good but long waits for routine services and difficulties in getting to see physicians are still common complaints.

To the extent that we develop close and effective working relations between consumers and doctors, we will have successful HMOs. Let me add, however, that people who are now being cared for by fee-for-service doctors have problems too: long waits for appointments, a doctor who doesn't give them enough time, a system that shunts them around from specialist to specialist without coordination or integration of care, and so forth.

People are not going to be totally happy with any system. You need one that is pointed in the right direction, and you must keep your eye on the big problems: the current system is going broke, it is not taking care of everybody, people are being destroyed financially by lack of insurance, and there's an enormous amount of waste, corruption, abuse, unnecessary duplication, and overhead. We must be willing to accept tradeoffs to get rid of all that and put in place a system that meets the basic requirements.

To get there, we have to move slowly and in stages. First, we must act immediately to control inflation or we'll be wiped out. However uncomfortable it may be, we must begin by freezing prices, insurance premiums, and payments to hospitals and doctors. In the long run, however, price control will not solve our problem because if you control prices service providers will protect themselves by providing more services. Still, we must do that now.

At the same time, we must begin to move the country in the direction that we want to go. Freezes won't generate the additional $35 billion to $80 billion a year needed to provide basic coverage for those not now covered. That will necessitate new taxes. "Sin" taxes could be a major source but wouldn't provide it all. You might also have to tax health care benefits above a certain amount. That would be even more unpopular than sin taxes, but you may have to do it. There may be other ways by which we will have to raise money.

I don't use an HMO today because of long personal relations with certain physicians. I get most of my health care from specialists I have known for years, and they are not in HMOs. If they were, I would not hesitate to join. If I had to participate in the system I described, it might disrupt my relations with some of my doctors but, then again, those specialists would probably join one HMO or another. The "superdocs" might want to stay out and could still earn their living, and I might have to pay extra for the privilege of staying with them. I would have to see who the HMO specialists were. After all, each field has more than one good specialist. I have my favorites because of longstanding personal contacts. It will take to the end of this decade or longer to reach a working equilibrium. Doctors, particularly those nearing the end of their careers, who have been practicing one way for a long time, are not likely to want to change, and they won't have to. But most of the young physicians coming along will be glad to accept the change.

As for the issue of medical malpractice insurance, we don't have an exact number for what it costs the country. Professional malpractice premiums are about $5 billion or $6 billion a year, and hospitals pay another few billion. That's about 1 percent of the total cost of today's health care. It's impossible to estimate how much "defensive medicine" adds to that. "Defensive medicine" is sometimes hard to define. It contributes something but it's not the most important cost by a long shot.

In well-run group practices there's a lot of internal monitoring and peer review, so that an incompetent or impaired physician is unlikely to go unnoticed. In a private solo practice, the doctor is not as directly accountable to anybody and if he or she is incompetent or impaired no one may know what's going on until something bad happens to a patient. Therefore, HMOs will run a lesser risk of malpractice, incompetence, physician impairment, and so on, and I suspect that their malpractice premiums will be much lower.

Nevertheless we ought to try to improve the current system through tort reform. We ought at least to look at a no-fault approach because the present system serves no one well except the trial lawyers. Only a minority of the damaged patients get compensated, and there is little evidence to show that this terribly expensive legal system discourages malpractice or improves the quality of health care. We have to do better. We should try to separate malfeasance, a professional issue that ought to be dealt with by professional peer review mechanisms, from maloccurrence. A maloccurrence that is not part of the natural history of the disease damages the patient whether there's been malfeasance or not. For example, a patient may receive the right dose of the right drug for the right indication and, because of an undetected sensitivity, still have a catastrophic reaction to the drug that causes permanent damage. Although nobody was at fault, if the patient is to be compensated for the tremendous economic and personal damage that he or she has suffered, under the present system it must be proven in court that somebody was responsible.

We can learn much from the experience, good and bad, in different health care systems—Canada's, England's, Germany's, Hawaii's, and Rochester's in New York—but in the last analysis, we have to develop our own system. We are a unique country with special needs, and we cannot simply transfer an existing system to the United States.

Part Five

CONFRONTING OBSTACLES AND SETBACKS

For some individuals the pathway to medicine is neither smooth nor trouble-free. Regrettably, the medical world has not lacked for prejudice in one form or another. For a long time women and racial minorities confronted major obstacles when they tried to make their way into the profession. The first story in this section is that of an elderly practitioner of family medicine whose career has been successful and fulfilling but who still rankles at indignities recalled. The second story includes encounters with malpractice litigation and conveys the impact of those experiences on a caring and talented physician. The third story tells how a personal illness can modify one's career directions in medicine.

In comparison to the vicissitudes experienced by other physicians, these examples illustrate more subtle trials, hurdles, and barriers. I've known doctors who were permanently confined to a wheelchair, whose dyslexia was so severe they had to go through medical school with virtually no sleep because each book had to be read two or three times, who had marked visual or hearing impairments, and who had to overcome the limitations of cerebral palsy. Courage, determination, and nobility are not confined to the patients. Sometimes an awareness of how other people have surmounted severe impairments or obstacles can help the rest of us to cope with the lesser hardships that intrude on our own lives.

Chapter 27

RACIAL BARRIERS

Dr. Walter C. Reynolds practices family medicine in Portland, Oregon. His story speaks for itself.

Walter C. Reynolds, M.D., Family Medicine,
Private Practice

I treat everyone who comes along and I see many people who are underprivileged and on welfare. They face multiple problems, and as I listen to these people I can't believe the extent of their troubles. . . . I could have gone in many wrong directions, but there was always a deep-seated feeling in me and my siblings of responsibility to our parents and family that kept us going in the right direction. That's part of how I got to medical school.

My decision to go into medicine began around 1936, during my sophomore year in high school. My family always felt that education was paramount and my older brother was an excellent student who helped guide me when I was more interested in sports than anything else. Around my sophomore year, I began to think about science, and medicine surfaced because I liked working with people.

I was born and raised in Portland, Oregon and educated in public schools. At that time, there was only one black physician in the whole state, Dr. Unthank, a fine family doctor in solo practice. When I sought counsel from my high school advisor, I was told there was not much point in thinking about medicine because there were essentially no black physicians in Oregon and I should not waste my time and energy. In those days, Oregon was very prejudicial in its patterns. I was irritated, frustrated, and concerned that someone should tell me this when I had expressed an interest, particularly when I knew that such counsel was not given to other students. It set a tone for me; I got angry about society's impact on me because I was black.

That experience helped motivate me. My brother, who experienced similar problems, went into physics and mathematics, eventually serving in the military. Then he joined the Naval Ordinance Depot in California, which played a large role in developing the Polaris missile. He experienced many of the frustrations of being black, such as never receiving the promotions he deserved on the basis of merit. It had a tremendous psychological impact on him, and at one time he was in psychiatric counseling; eventually, he made it.

My parents are wonderful people. My father was born out of wedlock in Macon, Georgia. He received a third-grade education and left home at age 15 after living through many oppressive problems. He falsified his birth date and got into the military. This gave him a nice hiatus for organizing his life, his concepts, his ideas about family life, and other things that served him and the rest of us well later on.

He settled in Portland in the early 1920s, worked as a railroad redcap, and eventually became a supervisor. He was firmly set on the value of education, not only for his own children (three boys and a girl) but for others. He encouraged many young people and gave them railroad jobs to help pay for their schooling. One of these individuals is now the editor of Portland's newspaper, *The Oregonian*. My father assisted in civil and legislative programs concerning Portland's social problems, and there were many.

Portland's liberal image was superficial. Because Oregon has had so few minorities, so much could be masked. My school was integrated, but there were only four blacks in it. Throughout my schooling here, there were signs all over the community saying "Whites Only." It was only a few years ago that the final discriminatory law was taken off the books. When I was coming along, things were really bad.

My father never made clear why he chose to live here except that he liked Portland. He never voiced regrets—he didn't look back.

Only with difficulty would he recount things that happened to him in the past. He was always positive in his attitude and in his approach. In spite of the environment and attitudes, he always told his family that these things are not right or just and that we should try to change them, but only by working within the legal parameters and framework.

Mother was equally intent on educating her children. She was from Minnesota. She moved to Idaho and met my father there when he was leaving the service. Then they moved to Portland. Their close family relationship helped us enormously. Like many black parents at that time, their message was to get an education to survive. The other message was that if you own land, they, the enemy, can't take it away from you.

Today those values are still there, but people are having difficulty understanding the need to pay the inner price and how to go about upholding them. It's difficult to describe. In my family practice, I treat everyone who comes along and I see many people who are underprivileged and on welfare. They face multiple problems, and as I listen to these people I can't believe the extent of their troubles. The problems repeat themselves over and over again. Portland is high in the drug trade, particularly marijuana, and it now has gangs raising havoc. All this makes it difficult to provide for children as my parents did. I had my problems coming up. I could have gone in many wrong directions, but there was always a deep-seated feeling in me and my siblings of responsibility to our parents and family that kept us going in the right direction. That's part of how I got to medical school.

In the 1930s, blacks could only get jobs related to service: railroad redcaps and porters, hotel maids, gatemen, and elevator operators. I could not get a job in a service station, or working behind the counter, or waiting on tables, or teaching, or working as a bank clerk. Because Dr. Unthank worked for the railroad and because so many of the black families were involved with the railroad, he had many black families as his patients. There were only 2000 blacks in Portland in 1935.

Dr. Unthank was from Kansas City and went to medical school for the first 2 years at Kansas City University. Those were the basic sciences years, and the third and fourth years were clinical. Because the idea of blacks working in the clinics examining females, and especially doing pelvic exams on white females, was unacceptable, at the end of his second year he was transferred to Howard Medical School, an all-black institution in Washington, D.C., for completion of his medical education.

He commented about that experience many times. Much like my father, although he appreciated the problems he always had a positive attitude. As a citizen of Portland, he was aggressive in promoting change. He was president of the Urban League and the NAACP. He belonged to many civic groups and city clubs, as I did when I eventually followed and emulated him. In his medical practice, he treated everybody who came along and that's why, coming back to my own practice, I have always done the same. His influence on me was great but indirect. Although I did not need to see him often as his patient, his presence in the community was significant to me. For a black physician to be able to function in the setting I've described took unusual ability and inner resources, and that impressed me.

My older brother, the one I described earlier, set an example for the rest of us. My younger brother has been active nationally and locally in the State of California and the County of Los Angeles. He taught for a while, became an administrator, and then handled grants in the university system, particularly those related to child health care centers. My sister is a graduate of the University of Oregon and works in the business world.

As blacks, we had no trouble getting into the educational system in Portland. There were so few of us in the whole state that it did not create problems. At first it was deceiving because it looked like the system treated us the same as everybody else. Then we began to perceive the subtle, and often not so subtle, impacts of what our whole society looked at in terms of ethnic groupings.

My advisor telling me not to think of medicine because I was black was just one of the signs of discrimination, but it hit real hard. When my older brother was told the same thing by his counselor, he cursed the man who said it and consequently got kicked out of school. After he was readmitted, his blackness was so restrictive that he was dreadfully frustrated and nearly didn't graduate from high school. He had good grades, but the English teacher didn't like him and tried to block his diploma because of a late final paper. When he submitted the required paper he was accused of copying it from a book. It became a real confrontation. My father had to go to the school and verify my brother's handwriting and verify that he did not do this sort of thing. Ultimately they gave him his degree and he went to the University of Washington, from which he graduated with a masters degree in physics.

Our counselors undoubtedly thought they were doing the right thing for us as black students. We couldn't get good jobs and we had to worry about earning enough for bread and butter because those were depression years. We couldn't even get into the trades. It wasn't until almost the 1970s that a black person could become a carpenter in Portland.

After graduation from high school I wanted to go to college but couldn't. My older brother was in college and the family had to help him, so I agreed to help support the family and my older brother. I worked as a redcap and did janitorial jobs. A year went by, school time approached again, and when it was a month away I realized that I hadn't saved any money. Finally, I told my mom and dad that I was going to school. My father didn't like that; it was the only confrontation I ever had with him. He said they couldn't afford to help me, but I told him that was okay, I would get a job at school and make it on my own.

The University of Oregon was in Eugene and my railroad pass got me there. I had saved $150 and I sold my saxophone for $25. I got a job hashing at one of the dormitories, corrected math papers, and did National Youth Administration work for 35 cents an hour. I even started playing basketball but I didn't receive a scholarship. Everything fell into place, and I took my subject material in premedicine even though I didn't dare to dream that it would lead to medical school.

After 3 years, World War II intervened. I took a summer course in civil pilots training and got my license between my sophomore and junior years, but I was turned down by the air corps because I did not have the necessary visual acuity. By then, I was eligible to apply to medical school, so I was headed either there or into military service. I applied to the University of Oregon Medical School even though no black had ever attended. I told myself that since the others who were in premed with me were applying, I would do the same. I did think strongly about going to a predominantly black medical school like Meharry or Howard if I was turned down by Oregon, but I concluded that I would just go into the service, complete my education there, and then probably reapply to medical school when I go out.

I went to Portland for an interview and met Dr. West, a biochemist and a person I will never forget. After the interview, I received a letter of acceptance. I couldn't believe it! I showed it to my mother and she just looked at me and blinked her eyes. I'd never even been in a hospital but I decided to go ahead. It was a unique experience to be the first black to be accepted. Then, later, I turned out to be the first black to graduate.

I had a hard time during the first couple of years. In fact, I had to leave because I didn't do well in my sophomore year. I failed a class and was about to repeat it, but I chose instead to take a break by joining the service and getting away for a while. The school told me that when I got out of the service I would have a place in the appropriate class.

I went to Fort Lewis for basic training and then applied to officer candidate school. I was accepted and called before an assignment board. I asked to go into the medical service corps, the chemical warfare service, or the corps of engineers, but they assigned me to infantry school at Fort Benning, Georgia. I was one of their 90-day wonders, and I became a first lieutenant in the infantry and ended up in the Philippines in 1945. By the time I got there, the atomic weapon had terminated the war. The services were segregated then, and originally I was headed for the 93rd Infantry Regiment, an all-black unit, for a big push on Japan. But with the ending of the war, I stayed in Manila and spent a year helping to deactivate the military complex there.

In the middle of that year I arranged for my return to medical school. Two weeks following my discharge, I entered the fall class. It worked out well. I repeated the second year and finished in 1949. Because Dr. Unthank had told me repeatedly about his experience in medical school and had advised me to expect the same treatment, as I reached the end of my sophomore year I was prepared to be asked to transfer to Howard. As it turned out, nothing was said to me, but I learned later that there was quite a debate about what should be done with me before they elected to let me continue. I appreciated and respected that. I know that several professors felt strongly that I should continue, and I'm sure they had to battle hard to make it happen; but it did, and I completed my medical school training in Oregon.

I didn't know what I was going to do with my medical career. For me, the effort of getting through one year, and then the next, and then the next, left me without a lot of interest in planning. I took one year at a time and wanted to get past the hurdles in front of me. I always felt that no matter what I would have to go to a black hospital like Harlem General for my first year of postgraduate experience. I didn't believe anything else would be open to me.

Then an interesting situation arose. That was 50 years ago, and there were no black members of the faculty. But I must say that I thought several members of the faculty were wonderful people; one was Dr. Warren Hunter, a pathologist. Bless his heart, I have never forgotten him. Through the years, he had helped Japanese and Chinese minority students to arrange for internships in the midwest. I was the first black but he offered me the same help. He was connected with a hospital in Des Moines and thought I would enjoy training there. I wondered what I would do there, never having been that far east, but I appreciated his interest, thanked him, and put that hospital on my list of places to visit.

I still had my railroad pass, so I took the train to visit a military hospital in San Francisco, and then I rode east to an all-black hospital in St. Louis that no longer exists. From there, I went to Des Moines to look at the hospital that Dr. Hunter had recommended. It was only out of courtesy to him—I had no intention of going there. I was hungry and wanted to get back to my family. By then I was married and had one youngster.

I married in 1944, when I left school and went into the service. My wife is from Seattle. We met because I saw her picture in the newspaper and was attracted to her. Through community interests in Portland I had developed a tie to the Urban League and had learned that her father was the executive secretary of Seattle's Urban League. I didn't particularly care to meet him, but she was very good looking and I made efforts to meet her. Due to my persistence, eventually we got married and stayed married until she expired in April of last year from lung cancer. She never smoked, and it was the last thing you'd think she would develop. We have two boys and three girls, and none is in medicine.

I visited Des Moines without my wife because of the expense. Life in medical school was a little threadbare. I paid my respects to Dr. Hunter's friends at the Broadlawns Polk County Hospital. Today it has a big family practice center. Back then, they had 10 residents, 10 interns, and a supervising resident from the University of Iowa Medical School. It was a very independent operation. The administrator was a charming, laid back, 85-year-old gentleman who knew Dr. Hunter well. He said that Dr. Hunter had sent students there and to a couple of the other hospitals in Des Moines, and he felt I might enjoy it there. I talked to the personnel and was favorably impressed. So I signed up on the spot, even before I got home. I thought it would be beneficial to have more time away from Portland. My wife was flabbergasted that I hadn't even asked her, but it turned out well. I was the first and only black there, but the people were warm and friendly and the situation fulfilled my expectations. Dr. Hunter was truly a marvelous person.

It was a wonderful year and I learned a lot. In the midwest at that time there was a shortage of physicians in the outlying community areas, and so you got to practice a lot of hands-on medicine. Our place was a rural community hospital a few hundred miles away from the University of Iowa Medical School in Iowa City. When I thought about what I wanted to do in medicine, the question of how to make a living for my family influenced me more than anything else because specialty training took a long time. Without it, you could still get into practice, develop your abilities, and do many of the interesting things you learned in internship. So my sights were turned away from a specialty. Had I gone to a hospital connected with one of the predominantly black schools, such as Howard, I would have gotten into a specialty because it was the trend to become whatever you could become. But as I finally finished my requirements and became a physician, the main battle I saw ahead was providing for my family.

During my internship, I worked under the auspices of an air force program because they paid $75 a month, an enormous salary then. As a result, I owed the air force 2 years of service when I finished. I did not mind that because I had my private pilot's license and they let me fly again. My wife agreed to the arrangement and after internship I went in as a first lieutenant. They sent me to Randolph Field School of Aviation Medicine and I became an aviation medical examiner. One year later, I became a flight surgeon and was stationed at Alison Air Force Base, in the middle of Alaska. I thought that, once again, they were persecuting me!

My wife and two children came with me, and we had 2 relaxing years. Mainly what I learned was how to survive. I ended up as the base flight surgeon, which was not much because it was a small base. I ran into a lot of interesting problems because I was the only black there. Then came the decision as to whether to make military service a career. They offered many inducements including a bump up to major. The military was finally desegregated. It would have been a worthwhile career, especially economically, but my experiences in the segregated infantry had left me resistant to the military approach. I was not very conformist and elected to leave the military.

I felt I need more training so I took a 1-year general rotating residency at the San Mateo Community Hospital in the Bay area in California, with thoughts of going into general practice in medicine and doing some surgery. Technically, I'm a fine surgeon, but when it comes to judgment, there may be question mark. As I see it, the question in medicine is always how competent you are in relation to what is available in your community. My one caution has been not to make mistakes, especially about what I can and can't do. When more appropriate help is available, it should be utilized. Maybe that's why I use a lot of consultation in my practice; I want the best for my patients. All this led me to general practice, which I enjoyed tremendously because it fulfilled my wish to work with people.

After the year in San Mateo, I considered the Bay area as a place to practice. It would have been lucrative, but even then, in 1953, the area was very crowded. I elected to return to Portland because I liked it and felt it offered an appropriate educational setting for raising my kids. I also liked Oregon's environment. I love the beaches and the mountains.

I joined Dr. Unthank for a couple of months, but it didn't quite work out and I headed out on my own. Just then, Dr. Joiner, another black doctor in Portland, moved to Seattle and I took over his office. My practice turned out to be like Dr. Unthank's, mixed but predominantly black. I started in 1954 and I've been practicing in the same building ever since. In time, I purchased it. Before I did, I thought about getting out of general practice and doing something else like psychiatry or public health. However, after 5 minutes of consideration I realized that I liked general practice and didn't want to leave it. Then general practice developed into the specialty of family practice, and I took my boards and became a fellow in the Academy of Family Physicians.

I belong to a couple of prepaid health groups, and in my office I see mainly families with a lot of children. I see newborns after delivery and follow them. I have an older practice in an urban center described as "relatively poverty stricken," but actually that community benefitted from Lyndon Johnson's Model Cities Program for urban renewal. I started a family practice residency program at our local general hospital and it functioned for 3 years. It was a good program that unfortunately was opposed by the hospital's medical director, an internist; eventually it wound down. It paid for itself and was one of the best things that ever happened to that hospital, but the medical director felt that family practitioners were a waste of time. He was determined to make his hospital a tertiary care center and saw very little role for family practice.

Internal medicine was the thing then, but our program put out good residents. We trained them to be like our faculty—family practitioners who did medicine, geriatrics, pediatrics, psychiatry, and some minor surgery in the office. We encouraged our graduates to do more extensive surgery only if the setting was appropriate and the need was there, as it was in Des Moines when I trained there. The key thing was judgment: what are the problems and when do you need help?

I've enjoyed my 40 years in practice immensely. I didn't pressure my five kids to go into medicine because I wanted them to decide for themselves what they wanted to do. My own experiences were not simple or easy. If they had wished to do what I did, they would have had to set a course and follow through. All of them have done well in other areas. The oldest is 42 and the youngest is 28. The oldest lives in Seattle where she is administrator for the county commissioner. The next one works here with AT&T, another is an investment entrepreneur, one is in fashion design in California, and another is with a New York computer firm. Two of my children did consider medicine and took college preparatory courses in math and science, but they didn't stay with it. Perhaps one day I'll ask directly why they rejected medicine. Maybe I transmitted some of the pressures of my experiences; it's hard to tell and it's always puzzled me.

I would not say that life is easier today for a black student coming into medicine than it was for Dr. Unthank or me. Perhaps the right term is "different." The pressure is still there. I am active in trying to get black students interested in our medical school here, but when I look at the tenured faculty I still see no blacks. After I was the first black to go through, there were no others for 15–20 years, until finally two students came in together. One is now an anesthesiologist and the other is in ob/gyn. According to them, their experiences in the institution were terrible.

The anesthesiologist was born here, and much of his perceptions depend on his individual exposures and feelings. When you look for oppressive situations, you must consider whether you are being oversensitive or even paranoid, and whether your perceptions are based on reality. You must guard against that kind of distortion and try to be conservative in your assessments. But even so, these things are real. What my dad and Dr. Unthank taught me was to understand that they occur and to react according to what I thought was right and appropriate. "They"—it is always the enemy out there— can throw all kinds of crap at you but you must sort that out and do what you feel you need to do with your own life. That's the way you live through that stuff.

After the anesthesiologist graduated, he went to California and did well. Over lunch, during a return visit 3 or 4 years ago, I asked him how he had felt as the second black in the history of the medical school. After 5 minutes of silence, he said, "It was the most devastating experience in my life. It was hell." For 1 hour, he reviewed his experiences in detail. They were similar to what I had lived through, but we had reacted differently. I will take a lot of crap, but I understand what's going on and don't mind expressing how I feel to anyone about what's appropriate or inappropriate. I will see the way society is at the particular moment, but I will not let in interfere with what I want to do. After everything my dad went through, he concluded with, "We live in the best country in the world, but if you're going to change things, go at it in the proper way."

In any event, my young colleague interpreted and reacted to his experiences in a different way from me. He had some personality problems of his own. When I had to leave school for a year I experienced stress, but I came back and spent an entire year in the class of the professor who had flunked me. Boy, did I look forward to sitting in the front row of his class and staring at him. He did bad things. He had an almost psychotic obsession with having students who weren't likely to make it come up in front of the class to present a paper while he degraded and denigrated them. When it was my turn, I realized what he was doing and gave a good paper, but I never forgot that. A Chinese student who failed that course and flunked school altogether told me later that he would never forget that class. My feeling was that if I couldn't make it on my own, then to hell with it. But I would do all I could do.

I was isolated and had to learn study techniques on my own. I worked hard but didn't have great study habits. When I came back to the school in my junior year, I encountered a clinical partner who was a wonderful guy and showed me how he prepared for exams. One day I mentioned a test that was coming up and he said, "Well, that's professor so-and-so, let's go to the fraternity and look at his old exams." "Old exams?" I said. "Yes," he answered, "they've got exams from way back." A light went on for me. After analyzing the old exams, he said, "Here are five logical questions for him to ask." So I went home and studied those subjects intensely and sure enough, four of the five were on the exam. I got an A and my partner got a B. Those kinds of incidents were interesting. Of course, I could not join the fraternity then, and there are no longer any fraternities.

In the medical school today each class has 100 students. There are two African students in the freshman class, two blacks in the sophomore class, two in the junior class, and one in the senior class. One of them, who is now a sophomore, worked in my office one summer taking histories and meeting patients. He was born and raised in Portland and went to an all-black university in another state. He is a very good student, an athlete, a good communicator, and interacts well with people. He is sensitized to problems related to minorities but well balanced in his outlook and concerns. When he returned here to go to medical school, he never anticipated the attitudes he would run into. It was a real cultural shock to be a black in that position and experience the ways people regarded him.

The oppressiveness was subtle and difficult to relate. The experience in the medical school is not as severe as it was in my day, but the problems are still there—you can't completely erase or change a community's character. Society changes very slowly. Because Oregon was once one of the most prejudiced states in the country, those things still crop up. Once they had the Klan here, and they isolated the Chinese and treated them like dogs. But there are certainly many good things about Oregon now, and you must keep that in mind when you try to influence black youngsters to get into medicine. That sophomore student has adjusted well and has avoided being oversensitive.

I work with the Oregon Community Foundation and have found

the board members to be fascinating. People involved with giving can be very pontificating because they are well off and see things differently from those who are struggling. Nevertheless, by and large these are fine individuals. One program that began here last year started in the east, where a wealthy person told an elementary school class that if the students kept up with their studies he would pay for their college educations. I talked to a man doing the same thing here and offered to try to interest young blacks in the lower grades in a career in medicine. There has been a decline in the number of blacks entering medicine, males in particular, and I want to help turn that around. That's what I want to do from now on, even though at 71 I'm still practicing and am busier than I was 30 years ago. We can change things by starting at the lower grades.

One-parent families need more attention and help from those with whom they can relate. With the Foundation we're getting medical students involved in community activity and arranging for them to speak to young students. This helps them and is an invaluable way of improving the image of physicians in this country.

Oregon has been a pioneer in reaching outlying areas such as Indian reservations and migrant labor camps, all of which have massive, deeply rooted needs, and we want the medical student in training to become more attuned to these needs. It's the same for the big city neighborhoods as well. In Portland, a group that's been working with youngsters has seen an enormous turnaround because many of these youngsters need help and guidance. You can improve the circumstances of many young people. Every young person whom you can help to get through high school should at age 17–19 experience an organized activity such as the Peace Corps, the Job Corps, or maybe military service. I hope this country will establish a general job corps that will put all kinds of students into the inner cities to provide help for the youngsters who have gone astray. If you do that, it will make an enormous difference even if it will not solve everything.

I told that sophomore medical student that he was wise to go to the medical school here because he wants to practice in Oregon and be part of the community. I told him that whether his experiences would lead to problems was up to him but that should not be a deterrent. Even though Oregon has many problems, it is a good place to live and raise a family. He would like to join me in my practice and I'm interested; however, by the time he finishes, I may or may not still be in this world, so timing is the issue. Also, medical graduates today want a setting that provides good financial resources, good training, and leisure time with the family. These are most likely to be found in a group practice like an HMO, which is where most of the trainees are going. Solo private practice will be fading out slowly.

I don't encourage my young friend one way or the other; he must evaluate things for himself. I did say that as he goes along, his feelings will undoubtedly change and so will health care delivery. Many aspects of practice are changing professionally, economically, and even socially for the individual physician. I'm thinking especially about the impact of computerization and the probability of our eventually having a nationalized health care delivery system.

We need basic medical care for everyone in this country, but achieving that will not be easy. It will mean public acceptance of changes in our thinking about how care is delivered. We must examine the long-term benefits of other health care delivery systems in countries like Canada and Britain, and adopt their good features. It's a massive problem with no simple solution, but eventually there must be bottom-line treatment for everyone in this country.

Everyone in Portland can get access to medical care, even the homeless people. They can go to the emergency rooms although the load there is tremendous. Of people needing care, about 30 percent have a job but can't afford insurance. They pay as they go, and because they often don't have enough cash their care is episodic. If they need extended care, their savings are eaten up. People on welfare get some basic care, and it's probably better than the episodic care and maybe even as good as what the rest of the people get, depending on who delivers it.

My practice is 30 percent Medicaid and Medicare. Minority people compose a small segment of the indigent population in Portland, but it is significant because there are about 30,000 in the state. The paper work is excessive, but a computer has helped enormously. If we ultimately have a national system, we will need electronic help for billing and record keeping to survive. Students should be taught to live with these things now.

This year, I'm president of the medical school's alumni association. After I was selected to be on the board, I spent several years migrating up the ladder and then automatically became president. If it means anything, I'm the first black, but I don't think about that anymore. Among other projects, I work with the dean to recruit more minority students, particularly blacks. The track record is not great, but it's not as poor as it was. It's been difficult for many reasons: the low number of applicants, stringent admission requirements, and a disinclination to use anything like affirmative action that could give someone an edge by considering abilities that would contribute to someone's performance as a medical student, physician, and person in the community.

I don't advocate a quota system, but these students can be looked at one way or the other, and we could accept more than we do. A young lady from Portland went to school here; did well academically; was active in the community, church, and sports; and then went through Meharry, a predominantly black college. She wanted to return and practice here where her family lived. She applied and interviewed well but was not admitted because of unacceptable MCAT scores. Nevertheless, she was accepted to at least five other medical schools, including University of Southern California, Washington, and Jefferson, to name a few. I had her visit with the dean and the admissions people here to describe how disappointed she had been and how much difficulty she had taking the MCAT. I told them I didn't intend to put them on the spot but that I wanted to show them that there were considerations beyond the MCAT. She did very well at Washington University in St. Louis and joined the navy because they had paid for her schooling. The last time I heard from her, she was over in the Gulf where she performed well. She's interested in internal medicine.

During her meeting here, I told them about other students whom they had turned down. One was the son of the medical school's affirmative action person. He was accepted to Columbia University in New York, finished there, and is now in a residency. The nephew of one of my patients was admitted to the University of Texas, took a residency there in orthopedics, and has since returned to Portland to set up a practice. There were a couple of others. The point is that if we don't look at a student totally and if we rely solely on MCAT scores, we will miss many good candidates. My message had an impact for a while and we picked up two or three students, but that has dwindled again. It seems to require constant effort to attract black students to medicine.

I hope that by the time my term is up, the medical school's administration will have achieved a more positive attitude. I also hope that the community program that guarantees a college education will generate a reasonably sized pool of Oregon students interested in medicine. It's a long-term project, but that's the way it has to be done. We'll also have to work on those who are now available from other states.

I have addressed white students in our medical school to tell them what it feels like to be at the receiving end of all this, and the message is usually well received. They are aware that it is not easy for any student to get into medical school. The makeup of the current entering class is fascinating. For the first time, there are more women than men and, by and large, they are a little older. The average age is 26, and one student is 45. The 95 people in the class were selected from 1064 applicants and 91 come from Oregon. There are 10 Asian students, 2 African-American students, and 1 Hispanic, so there's been some effort. This was a tough class to get into, and you can see the problem blacks have in fighting more competitive admissions, especially when they come from a state that has so few blacks to begin with.

I encourage minority students to concentrate first on getting into medical school and then dealing with the realization that the future holds many different possibilities. Any new medical student— black, white, or otherwise—should understand that with time he or she will develop interests in many areas. For selfish and personal reasons I encourage them to go into family practice medicine.

It can be a gratifying area, but in my time it has developed into a specialty and has acquired limitations. Some programs do not include obstetrics, and that's a loss because then you don't experience what it means to start a family. I don't deliver babies any longer, but I did when I was first in practice. I also did a little surgery and saw patients at all age levels. That was general practice in the true sense of the word. Today family practice does much of this, but it has been modified by educational and social settings. In larger cities, where there are surgeons by the dozen, you must be careful about what you do. If you make errors, you're going to have problems, so you gradually narrow things down. Today none of my peers does obstetrics; there are too many problems, too much time is involved, and malpractice insurance costs are enormous. The same goes for surgery. I assist at surgery with all my patients, but I do not do the surgery. I'm a primary care physician, almost like an internist. Basic procedures I once learned like spinal taps and paracenteses have gone to the highly specialized. We're down to general family practice with a lot of screening, psychiatric consultation, family problems, and environmental, general health, and public health concerns.

If I were starting out today, I would think more about a specialty such as surgery or ob/gyn, and I think that is what's happening to family practice. Many students are not leaning toward family practice, but for certain individuals it is ideal because it offers an entry to all areas of medicine. The programs vary depending on the community's needs. Iowa, where I trained, was an agrarian community where graduates went to the boondocks and did everything. The university here is experiencing that same need in smaller communities, and they are training their family practice residents accordingly. So if you can show students that the nature of the field changes from place to place, you will increase the family practice population.

My office is in the core of the inner city, near a big teaching hospital. I have about five patients in the hospital each day for whom I care, and I work in my office through the day until 6 or 7 o'clock at night, just seeing patients. Though my patient population is predominantly black, it is mixed. Oregon is not a very potent state economically, although our unemployment level is a little less than the national average.

I find myself working most of the time. My hobbies are my family and trying to work with the computer. I'm an avid basketball fan and I've gone to Blazer games since they started. When I watch those great athletes, I dream that, gee, maybe one day I'll have the potential.

I encourage medical students to develop a good overview of where they're going and to assess the fields in which they might be interested. That opportunity comes largely in the third and fourth years. They should orient themselves to the changing aspects of medicine, including technology. Before long, invasive tests will be minimal. A patient will go into an MRI-like module and undergo a total analysis. Medicine will change by the time students get out, and it's hard to appreciate what's happening when you're in the middle of it. Yet it's always wise to be positive about what you do. I'm a little cautious about what's going to happen, but even at age 71 I'm optimistic. We live in exciting times. There's been nothing like it in human history.

Chapter 28

MALPRACTICE LITIGATION

Dr. Murray Pendleton is a retired pediatrician. During his active professional career he worked in a practice associated with Boston teaching hospitals, was in private practice in a small community on Cape Cod, and, after experiencing two malpractice lawsuits, went to work in a state hospital for rehabilitation and chronic care.

Murray Pendleton, M.D., Pediatrics, Private Practice

I liked the idea of being able to follow the baby through gestation and as a newborn—a continuum of care.

I was born in Boston and brought up in Waterbury, Connecticut. For the past 32 years I have lived in Falmouth, Massachusetts. I started thinking about going into medicine at the age of 6 when I had a stiff neck with a fever and no paralysis. It was labeled polio and even though I wasn't very sick, I was hospitalized. That hospitalization turned out to be a pleasant experience with angels of mercy all around me. Subconsciously I came to feel that practicing medicine would be a wonderful thing to do. When I was 9, my favorite cousin called me a "natural doctor," and from then on I seemed to be heading into medicine.

I landed in Harvard Medical School by virtue of good luck. My college experience was cut short by the war and so I ended up with mainly premedical training rather than an education. In medical school my role models were primarily clinicians and I decided that I would be one of them. I am certain that among those people who become doctors some are born to be surgeons and some to be primary care physicians. The two groups think differently. A surgeon needs the capacity for black-and-white thinking and the ability to make a decision and act quickly. The surgeon can't go back and undo what he or she has done, whereas the family physician, the pediatrician, or the internist usually has the opportunity to think at greater length and then take action. Because I am not a black-and-white thinker, I felt that I was unsuited for surgery. I admired pediatricians; many of them were what I wanted to be like. I didn't have the patience for psychiatry although it was my best subject in medical school; I wanted results.

Trauma never interested me but naturally occurring disease did, and so during my clerkships I decided to aim for internal medicine. It was close to family practice, and that was what I had in mind. I applied to the Mass. General and the Brigham, but I didn't get into either one and was devastated. Fortunately, Sidney Farber, a professor of pathology at Children's Hospital in Boston, came to my rescue and arranged for me to spend 16 months as a resident in pathology at Children's. I had an absolutely terrific time. Even though I enjoyed working with the people in his department and liked Dr. Farber, while I was there I had enough exposure to clinicians to conclude that I really wanted to go into clinical pediatrics.

After that, I did a 2-year stint in the navy as a pathologist, radiologist, obstetrician, and pediatrician. Then I applied for pediatrics training at Children's and was admitted. My residency began rather traumatically because it was in the middle of a severe polio epidemic, but my training time at Children's was the high point of my professional life. My first assignment was doing dozens of lumbar punctures a day for outpatient polio screening. I had a terrific senior resident who became a good friend. During my training, most of what I learned above and beyond hands-on experience came from my fellow residents and from my responsibilities for teaching students.

At that time we knew that polio was caused by a virus, but there was no prevention or cure, and the clinical tools we had were merely supportive. We dealt with it somehow. Polio was a cloud over our professional lives as it must be with AIDS today. It's tough for a physician's horizon to be filled with such an epidemic of growing dimension. We need another miracle.

In 1952, after my 3 years of clinical pediatric training, I went into clinical practice with a group based at the Boston Lying-In Hospital and at Children's. We focused on newborns—problems related to their maturity and to their respiratory systems. I practiced with the group for 6 or 7 years doing general pediatric practice, including house calls. It was exciting to see youngsters in their home. I had a little microscope and did white counts at the bedside. We did a lot of hospitalizations but not as many as are done now because those were less litigious times. I taught neonatal pediatrics and enjoyed that tremendously. You didn't have to be as smart then as now; we weren't all involved in blood gases.

I did clinical research related to eye movements in the newborn. With a radiologist I did a combined study on respiratory distress syndrome. Then the head of our group obtained a multihospital NIH grant to study cerebral palsy, and I gave up the general pediatrics practice to become the deputy director of his study. I continued a neonatal practice within the hospital and became a clinical neonatologist. I enjoyed the clinical work, but I was spending a great deal of time in administration without being a very good administrator. I also monitored obstetricians for the Massachusetts Medical Society to tell them where they had gone wrong in caring for newborns, mainly with regard to excessive anesthesia or analgesia, and that made me somewhat unpopular. Eventually I realized that I was ready for a change.

I decided to take an obstetrics residency and see for myself where the newborns came from. It was a crazy plan but seemed to make sense at the time. It was a sudden decision—I woke up one morning and said, "This is it." I was 38, married, and had five kids. I was accepted at Albert Einstein and got a 4-year NIH grant to train to be an obstetrician and a pediatrician, that is, a perinatologist, although the term was not yet in use. At that time, obstetricians would deliver a baby and turn it over to the pediatrician. Many of them wouldn't bother to find out what happened to the baby; their concern was the mother. My concern was the baby.

I became involved in a research project at Einstein and I delivered hundreds of babies. After a year, I realized that I couldn't maintain my schedule and have a family of five kids and a wife living in Massachusetts. I commuted back and forth every other weekend and found the logistics to be terribly stressful. Also, the research was unproductive. After 6 months of doing deliveries and assisting

with surgical procedures, I decided that a year of concentrated obstetrics was enough to permit me to begin a combined obstetrics
and pediatrics practice. Unfortunately, I didn't appreciate that a pediatrician who practiced obstetrics without having boards in obstetrics was setting himself up for problems. But I liked the idea of
being able to follow the baby through gestation and as a newborn—
a continuum of care.

I left Einstein and came to Falmouth to do obstetrics and pediatrics. I didn't go back to Boston because it wouldn't have been appropriate for a non–board-certified obstetrician to do obstetrics there.
Instead, I went to the equivalent of an underserved or rural area.
There wasn't even a hospital here yet. I felt that I knew more about
pregnancies and deliveries than perhaps most general practitioners
did.

I spent a straight year on call. I had a lot of support and referrals,
and it worked out well. It proved physically grueling. Being up all
night delivering a baby and then having office hours throughout the
next day became tolerable when another pediatrician came to town
and we covered for each other in pediatrics. Then some competent
obstetricians moved here who proved to be understanding and helpful. I could call on them to do sections and what-have-you. But then
came the lawyers and eventually I became disenchanted and gave
up obstetrics. I was delivering about 100 babies a year, and generally
there is a 1 percent likelihood that something will go wrong. I was a
sitting duck for a law suit, especially since I was not fully creden-
tialed in obstetrics. As it turned out, I went through two malpractice
suits, one for obstetrics, and one for pediatrics.

In the obstetric suit the patient was a primiparous patient who
was doing well and who had electrodes in place to follow fetal heart
patterns. At one point the fetal heart developed an irregularity that
lasted for a short while and then disappeared. I didn't act. Then,
when it reappeared, I tried a midforceps delivery but the baby was
hung up. I called in a fine obstetrician who arrived within 15 minutes and he did a forceps delivery. Although the baby survived, it
was damaged neurologically. I'm certain the damage had occurred in
utero.

Sadly enough, the mother kept coming back to me with the newborn and it was obvious that development wasn't going well at all.
One morning, after a year had passed, I read in the local newspaper
that I was being sued. I don't know how the paper learned about it

even before I got the letter from the lawyer. He was something of a celebrity who had written a book that had been made into a movie, *The Verdict*, with James Mason and Paul Newman. The parents had reason to sue; there had been a bad outcome. They had had an obstetrician with 1 year's training and during the emergency a specialist had to be called in. On the other hand, I did a reasonably good job taking care of the newborn; I don't think it would have lived if I hadn't given it such care. The baby was compromised to begin with, and in all probability the damage had occurred before delivery. No one can say for sure if it could have gone differently, but I can't help wondering if things would have gone better had the delivery been effected immediately.

I was about 5 years into the combined practice when this oc-curred, and I decided right then and there—no more obstetrics. I completed my responsibility to the patients I was taking care of prenatally, delivered them, and then didn't take any new obstetric patients. The litigation took 2 or 3 years and it made me doubt that I had made the right decision about obstetrics. I had been too sure of myself when planning my career change; I had thought I was pretty good, but maybe I was not that good. I felt very sympathetic to the parents for their misfortune. My insurance company settled the case out of court. I had a lot of support from the medical community. A leading obstetrician in Boston who reviewed all maternal deaths and perinatal problems for the state medical society was prepared to testify on my behalf. He wrote a wonderful review of the case and I never heard anything negative about my actions from my peers here.

Before the obstetrics suit, I'd had one in the pediatric part of my practice while I was still in the combined practice. A 4-month-old infant who was suffering from several days of intractable massive diarrhea was brought in from a small town on the Cape. The local doctor had said he couldn't cope with the situation any longer and had sent the child to a community hospital on the Cape. In the emergency room there they said they couldn't deal with the problem either and they referred her to the emergency room here. I happened to be on call for the emergency room and saw the moribund baby, who was then completely dried out. This was before the days of oral rehydration. I didn't think she was going to live.

I treated her with intravenous fluids and she came around, but she remained extremely lethargic. The lab work revealed a hyperna-tremic type of dehydration with a very high blood sugar. I decided to give the baby a small amount of insulin in addition to the fluids and she had a seizure, which she came out of. Since then research has shown that hyperglycemia can be a factor with hypernatremic dehydration, but I couldn't have known it then. I can't help but feel that the small amount of insulin I administered might have contributed to the seizure. That baby has since become a teenager who has, I gather, some neurologic damage. After the acute situation, I referred the child to a neurologist at the Mass. General. The specialist followed up neurologically and I continued to give general care for 6 or so months, whereupon I received notice that I was being sued. The neurologic outcome was being attributed to the insulin I had administered. Although a chain of doctors had been involved before me, I was being blamed for the outcome. Incidentally, the parents' lawyer was the same one who later was involved in my other lawsuit.

I don't know whether I bear any responsibility for the outcome, but I feel that I shouldn't have given the insulin because the child did not have diabetes. Two nationally known pediatricians supported me fully, as did the community, but then again it wasn't likely that people would seek me out to tell me I was a lousy doctor. The matter was never argued in court because there had been a recent pediatrics suit in another town in Massachusetts and the award to the parents had been something like $10 million. My insurance company settled in a hurry.

The case's effect on me was delayed for 2 or 3 years, but it led to my decision to leave pediatrics practice. I became a bit paranoid. Although by and large my patients' parents had been my friends, I began to think of them as potentially litigious enemies. I lost the spark and no longer enjoyed taking care of patients and talking to parents. So I gave up practice. I don't know how much was burnout and how much was due to the law suits. Back when I was teaching medical students in Boston, I always told them that a terribly important part of any illness is the family's feeling of guilt and that one of the duties of a pediatrician is to assume their guilt to help them. Maybe that's not such a good idea in this day and age. Someone is going to turn around and bite you.

When I decided that I'd had it with practice and announced as much at a staff meeting, I had absolutely no plans. I was 55 with a wife, five children, and no independent means. I've never been poor, but I've never been rich. I figured I could always do something, even if I had to flip hamburgers for a living. My wife, who had been a social worker, wrote to old friends and told them that I needed a job, but nobody responded. Then she and I went to a medical meeting where we ran into an old friend. At one time he had wanted to join me in practice here, but the other pediatrician in town had said that there wasn't enough pediatrics activity for three.

My wife went up to him in tears and asked whether he had a job for me. "It just so happens, I do," he said. He was the chief of staff at Lakeville Hospital, an excellent state institution for rehabilitation and chronic care, half for children and half for adults. It was for all comers. Those who weren't indigent paid. My friend was looking for a director of pediatrics and so in 1978, a short time after I'd quit practice, I started at Lakeville and I went on to spend a wonderful decade there.

I provided hands-on care for neurologically damaged babies and children who could not be cared for at home. It was fascinating. In a way I suppose it was restitution for the neurologic damage that I may or may not have caused others, but that wasn't why I went there. I went because I was going to work with someone I liked, I was going to do pediatrics, and I would not have to buy malpractice insurance. It was far from a nine-to-five job and for the first 5 years I stayed over 1 or 2 nights a week. I found it better than practice, largely because the parents were especially grateful for what you did for their children.

To live with yourself in practice you have to be egotistical enough to think you're pretty darn good. You sit on your throne in your own empire and everybody comes to you for the healing hand. That does something to your ego; and if you lose a little of it, you can't be entirely giving without getting something back in return. When you're practicing you need strokes every now and then, but now I don't care any longer.

I don't think medicine should be a business. I was never happier than when I was doing a good job for patients, collecting a paycheck at Lakeville, getting my professional insurance covered, and not thinking about money. If you have to cut short the time you spend with patients because you need to see more patients in order to make a living, that's not right. Many doctors in private practice are forced into that situation not because they are greedy but because limited and complex third-party payment schedules favor procedural over cognitive medicine and force them into it.

When I started practice in Boston, we used to say that we would take care of your baby from birth to age 1 year, and that it would cost a specified amount of money no matter how many visits we had to make, no matter what we had to do. If a child had to be hospitalized, that would be an additional cost. Then it became so much per visit. Then Medicaid arrived and it became so much for a hematocrit, so much for a urinalysis, so much for other tests, and so much for shots rather than adequate compensation for time spent with patients. To add it all up, your nurse had to spend most of the time handling money matters.

I don't know what's coming down the road, but I think we should have national health insurance. I was a government employee providing care and I loved it. You can maintain the quality of care by monitoring the kind of people you recruit to those institutions. You need to select nurses, doctors, and support people who are dedicated and who love kids. I hope that is the kind of person who will go into health care, but I don't know how to evaluate it objectively and choose accordingly. The whole matter of financing in medical care is beyond me, but I can't see how it could be any worse than having the insurance companies running medicine.

The whole diagnostic-related group (DRG) thing has sort of grown out of this. A physician often has to answer to someone who is sitting behind the desk in an insurance company and is making what should be a medical decision on behalf of an individual who can't afford to pay more than what the insurance covers. That is managed care, and it's going to be the doctors who are managed by the insurance company. If the management were done by a physician, who could relate physician-to-physician, it could work. We would need that in a national health program too. Dealing with a nonphysician gatekeeper can be a problem. In an insurance company system, the best interest of the patient runs up against the best interest of the budget. I suppose the same conflict of interest arises in the government arrangement because in effect the government is a business. So I guess gatekeepers are necessary, but we need knowledgeable and empathetic ones who also understand costs.

I retired from Lakeville when I was 65. At the time my wife had lymphoma invading her spine and pressing on the cord. She was operated on in Boston by a superb surgeon. He scraped all the tumor out, and she had radiation and chemotherapy. In the preradiation phase she discovered her own breast tumor. She had an infiltrative carcinoma of the breast and got radiation for both lesions. Fortunately, there was no node involvement. Although she realizes that whenever one talks about cancer it has more to do with remission than cure, the important thing is that she's feeling fine right now.

At first my wife and I did things around the house, although I'm not very good at it. After things settled down, I went back to work at Lakeville for a year and a half because they needed me to fill in for someone, but now I am completely and really retired. I'm trying to learn to be a grandparent to nine grandchildren and it isn't all that easy; it takes work. Last year, I joined the senior section of the American Academy of Pediatrics and they made me secretary–treasurer of the section. That's been sort of fun. Once again, my wife got me into something that is interesting, a group called Generations United that meets every spring in Washington. One issue being addressed is the role of grandparents in the care of "crack babies" because the mothers usually take off. It's not that demanding and I don't do that much, but it's exciting.

If I were starting all over again today, I would go into medicine again. None of my children did—I guess in part because they lived through my law suits. That affected the entire family. Without question, I would go into pediatrics again, but I'm not sure what aspect.

How do you choose your way in medicine? You have to know yourself and your talents. I have no idea what percentage of my medical school colleagues followed through with the decisions they made by the end of the second year of medical school. I do know about one; he said he went into medicine to make money, and he did. I hope he has been happy with his practice.

In the senior section of the Academy of Pediatrics residents meet with over-the-hill pediatricians like me who pass on our experiences. The same kind of program might help in medical school and even in residency training programs. Experienced, retired physicians could be useful to students and teachers in an informal way. After our meeting last spring, we met with residents who seemed genuinely excited to talk to their predecessors and to find out what we have done right or wrong. There's value in sharing this experience.

Chapter 29

PERSONAL ILLNESS

Although Dr. Ganson Purcell exhibited some interest in administration early in his career, it was not until his rheumatoid arthritis became severe enough to interfere with his surgery that he moved toward managerial work and curtailed the scope of his clinical activities. When this interview was conducted, he was chief of staff of the hospital of the University of Massachusetts Medical Center in Worcester, and professor of obstetrics and gynecology in the center's medical school. Three years later, he left to become chairman/director of the Department of Obstetrics and Gynecology for the St. Francis Hospital and Medical Center and the Mt. Sinai Hospital, in Hartford, Connecticut. He also holds the position of associate chairman of obstetrics and gynecology at the University of Connecticut and he continues to see patients with gynecologic problems on an outpatient basis.

Ganson Purcell, M.D., Obstetrician/Gynecologist; Department Chairman; Community Teaching Hospital

I must say, though, that when I saw the chair of ob/gyn at Tufts about a teaching role, he asked me something that planted a seed in my mind: "Do you feel with your background that you will be happy in the practice of general obstetrics and gynecology for 35 years?"

I sort of backed into medicine. I always had an interest in things medical and can remember aunts and uncles saying when I was a child that I would make a good doctor. When I went off to college my initial major was political science. Toward the end of my sophomore year, when I began to think seriously about what I wanted to do, nothing jumped out and grabbed me. Then I realized that I enjoyed the few science courses I had taken and began to think about medicine. I took a summer course in organic chemistry, got my B, and changed my major to biology.

Because I am a sailor, I spent my summers during high school and college working in shipyards and places like that. One summer I worked part time and went to secretarial school because, having decided to go into medicine, I realized I was going to have to take notes very fast. I considered volunteering at a hospital, but somebody in medicine advised me to do what I wanted to, which was to see what I could of the world. Looking back, I think that medical volunteer work would have been a better idea.

It's not abundantly clear to me how I crystallized my decision for medicine, except that I liked people and didn't like being ill myself. I'd had a wonderful pediatrician who was right out of a Norman Rockwell painting, something of a role model. I finished college, applied to medical school, and was accepted by Columbia. Since the doctors I knew were practitioners, I assumed that I would be one too.

The summer after our freshman year was my only free one, and I decided to get a feeling for what people did in medicine by obtaining a grant to work in the coagulation lab at Columbia's hospital. Back then, in the mid-1950s, coagulation was the province of obstetrics and gynecology because of bleeding episodes in the first and third trimesters of pregnancy. The internists hadn't gotten into it yet, and open heart surgery was just a gleam in somebody's eye.

That experience stimulated my interest in obstetrics and gynecology. I was exposed to the many clinicians who were interested in what was going on in our lab, and they were receptive to my questions. I went through the third-year clerkships and my decision came down to ob/gyn or internal medicine. I took three internal medicine electives at Bellevue Hospital, which captivated me, and I went to see the chief of the Columbia division at Bellevue to discuss my choice of a direction in medicine. He suggested that if I was uncertain I should take a rotating internship.

That was valuable advice, and today I regret the dissolution of the rotating internship. It gave a good opportunity to pick and choose among medical fields because one could almost design one's own curriculum. Rotating internships were eliminated, I believe, because people came to feel that if you're going to specialize, you had better start right away. Today there still exists the "transitional year," which has the complexion of the rotating internship. Other reasonably enlightened disciplines have built into their first year what they call a mixed program. For instance, many ob/gyn programs have a significant section of internal medicine, but by then you've committed yourself to obstetrics and it's not really a sampling experience. That's why the rotating internship was so helpful.

I did mine at a general community hospital in Seattle, Washington. I chose the west coast after working one summer in the Idaho woods where I became enamored with the Pacific Northwest. I was married after my first year in medical school, and my wife, who was from the east, was willing to sample the northwest.

When I got my internship appointment in the spring of my senior year, I interviewed in the ob/gyn department at Columbia and I went to Seattle knowing I had a residency lined up back home. Today you are pressed to make an early commitment to your field, and that is one of the unfortunate aspects of what I call compression in medical education. When I first came to UMass, students could take basic clerkships in either the third or fourth year. Not infrequently, one of them would come to me at the end of the fourth year saying, "I love the ob/gyn clerkship, but I've applied for a residency in pediatrics. What should I do?"

It was difficult to help them; some had already been accepted into a program. Even in our own ob/gyn residency program some residents decided after several months of the first year that it wasn't what they wanted and left in search of something else. To me this reflects the unfortunate pressure that is placed on students to make up their minds. It is somewhat helpful to have put the core clerkships into the third year so a student can sample them before applying for a residency. Also, the deadline for residency application was pushed back 6 to 8 weeks, and that has helped too. But students are still pushed.

I have another partial solution to the pressure problem, one that is reflective of my own career. When the Cuban missile crisis erupted in October 1962, I was 4 months into my internship. Like many young physicians in the country, I was drafted into the service. Although I had to delay my residency, I found the 2 years in the military a wonderful and valuable experience. I was a physician on a submarine and I became schooled in respiratory physiology and deep submergence problems. Military or public service can give people time to reflect before making a choice that might necessitate backtracking later on. Revitalizing the National Health Service Corps would be a good idea. It would bring care to underserved areas and address some of our national problems.

By the time I got my summer job in Columbia's ob/gyn department, my interests had begun to focus on the management of medical problems, on surgery, which I liked, and on delivering babies, which I loved. I also knew that I didn't want to work in fields like pathology and radiology and be removed from patients. I see internal medicine and surgery as complementary rather than antagonistic. When I counsel students considering ob/gyn, I caution them to avoid a misimpression during their undergraduate clerkship. Because we teach in an institutional setting, we plug students into the labor and delivery suite or the operating room, where they hold retractors, do exams under anesthesia, and do a history and physical. We leave out the reality that the practice of ob/gyn is an office-based discipline.

From my clinic work at Columbia, I learned that I liked the one-on-one interaction in the office, in other words, the counseling role. I also liked the thrill of delivering a baby and the discipline of surgery. When it all came together in one package, I thought it was terrific. My residual indecision about whether to go into internal medicine derived from my exciting experience at Bellevue with the kind of patients we saw there and the enthusiasm of the staff. However, when I did my rotation in medicine during my internship, I wound up managing medical problems that lacked dramatic change and realized that I wanted a discipline that provided rapid change and immediate gratification. Yet I liked seeing patients on a continuing basis, and the blend of these two aspects was what made obstetrics and gynecology right for me.

I also liked the policeman–fireman aspect. You sit around, wait for things to happen, and then go at a great pace. Still I appreciate the need to order one's personal and family life, and obstetrics and gynecology can accommodate successfully. As in other disciplines, more and more obstetrician–gynecologists are going into large groups, where one has time on call and time off. That goes a long way toward addressing the problem.

When I was drafted during my internship, I deferred the ob/gyn residency, finished my internship, and then spent 2 years in the navy. That tour of duty allowed me to practice some medicine and apply my research background. When I went in, there was a concern that prolonged submergence might cause coagulation problems among the sailors and I was able to show that this was not so. I found that as a leftover from the days when the diesel subs were very noisy, it was traditional to carry big bottles of APC tablets that contain aspirin. It turned out that some sailors took too much aspirin and that produced their coagulation problems. At that time people in medicine were beginning to discover the role of aspirin as an anticoagulant. I was pleased to be able to use my background to make a useful contribution. If submergence had been producing the coagulation changes, the navy would have had a serious problem.

I considered staying in the military because I was offered an ob/gyn residency with the proviso that I pursue the formalization of the specialty of submarine medicine. I decided not to because the young people have all of the fun in military medicine. The older you get in the military, the more administrative you become, and I didn't think that was for me. Ironically, that is what I do now.

So I entered my ob/gyn residency and a short time later the head of the coagulation lab left. The chairman of ob/gyn told me to take over the lab while doing my residency. I tried to decline the honor but to no avail. Fortuitously, a young man who had completed his ob/gyn residency at another institution wanted graduate training in coagulation and came on as a fellow. I was the titular head of the lab and he was its functional heart and soul. I wrote the new and renewal research grants and the progress reports.

I had to come to grips with a major issue for a doctor contemplating an academic career. If you try to be the mythical quadruple threat—practitioner, researcher, administrator, and teacher—however competent you may be, you will be stretched too thin and never handle any one of the areas well. I finally decided that what I did best was to treat patients, that I would not pursue research, and that I would try to keep on teaching. So at the end of my residency, I joined two men in private practice near Boston and took a part-time teaching appointment at Tufts Medical School.

My first child was born when I was in the service and the second after I was in residency for a year. I worked hard during the residency and gave it a lot of my time. I chose to believe that it did not take a toll on my growing family. I reasoned that once I went into practice with an established group, there would be time for family and personal pursuits. It worked out very well and I loved it. I must say, though, that when I saw the chairman of ob/gyn at Tufts about a teaching role, he asked me a question that planted a seed in my mind: "Do you feel with your background that you will be happy in the practice of general obstetrics and gynecology for 35 years?" As I became involved in hospital affairs and an officer of the medical staff, I found that I had a serious interest in administration.

After I had been in practice for 9 years, a personal health problem intervened. I had developed rheumatoid arthritis in high school. I'd been aware of it earlier, during residency but it became severe enough to cause difficulty in performing surgery. My rheumatologist, who had been trying to manage the disease with gold and steroids, advised me to consider giving up surgery and making changes in my professional life.

Having kept a hand in teaching, and having developed an interest in administration, I reviewed my options and considered going back to academic medicine. Not too long after, I was recruited by the University of Massachusetts Medical Center to help establish the ob/gyn department and be its vice chairman. I said that I would teach, practice ambulatory gynecology, and serve as an administrator, but that I would not pursue research or perform surgery. As a fledgling institution, its strategy for the development of the department was to address teaching and practice first and to build the research program later. My skills were consonant with what was needed right away and we went ahead.

I remained vice chairman for 3 years and became more involved in the entire institution's administrative pursuits. I helped to develop a day surgery program and to revamp the ambulatory care programs. In time I was invited to serve as liaison between the administration and the medical staff by being chief of staff of the medical center's hospital, and I've been in the job for 11 years.

By and large, the position's gratifications predominate—mainly because I have time for ob/gyn and can still pursue my practice. I learned how to do administrative work largely from on-the-job training but I have found it rewarding because I get to interact with many people and do different things. Because of my rheumatoid arthritis, I don't deliver babies or do surgery. I made a transition to ambulatory work where I treat mainly medical gynecologic problems. In addition to the reproductive age population, I have a special interest in pediatric adolescents and the menopausal age groups. I have found my role in medicine. I can't say whether I might still be in private practice if my rheumatoid arthritis had not gotten worse, but I can look back without regrets. What I do is exciting; I've molded a career with many interesting ramifications.

I don't think going into administration is a waste of training if you don't remove yourself completely from the clinical environment. We need physicians behind desks because, by dint of their training and experience, they are better prepared to make important administrative policy decisions. To be an effective administrator, I need to maintain contact with clinical practice; it makes me more confident about my administrative decisions and helps me to retain respect and credibility among my peers. The crux of administration is helping others to make decisions rather than sitting as a committee of one and making the decisions alone. If I had to do that I'd make many wrong decisions, but facilitating decision making among thoughtful people is a valuable contribution.

Changes and trends pervade my clinical field. In the future, the obstetrician–gynecologist is going to become less of a specialist and more of a generalist with an expanded role as a primary care physician. Operative gynecology is decreasing because we manage more problems medically. We are seeing much less major operative gynecology than we saw a decade ago, and more and more is being performed on an outpatient or office basis. Over the last decade, the number of ob/gyns who include obstetrics in their practice had dropped. Among the reasons are limitations in manpower and the professional liability crisis. Babies are being delivered by a shrinking cadre of obstetricians and by midwives. My crystal ball says that in the not-so-distant future there will be groups of four to six obstetrician–gynecologists with two or three doing the obstetrics together with a complement of midwives. It's a social reality and a tenable model that will make for good obstetrics.

The country's female population is large and increasing. The population segment that will experience significant growth in this next decade is women over 45. There will be more demands made of the obstetrician–gynecologist to address the problems of women in the menopause. We are considering restructuring our residency and undergraduate curricula to emphasize a greater role in primary and preventive care. It is important for students planning to enter the field to be aware of the potential changes. Also, the curricula in family practice and internal medicine should be modified to include a larger quotient of gynecology.

It is advisable for a student to enter medical school determined to keep options open, to maintain an interest in everything that is offered, and to use initiative in seeking alternatives. For as long as possible, particularly if you feel undecided, keep the choices open and try not to feel pressured. Think about taking a quantum of time—even as long as a year—to pursue something even if you might abandon it after the year. Do not feel that you have to run headlong into something. Although a year may seem long while you're in training, when you look back later it isn't a very long time.

Managing the pressure of having to pay off education loans that can amount to $60,000 to $100,000 poses an awful dilemma. I would change the system so you don't have to begin repaying the debt until you complete your training. I would allow for a testing year during the training period for trying out a discipline.

I don't have reservations about advocating a career in medicine. We have a malaise in medicine now, and appropriate adjustments are needed. As a society we place too much value on health care and not enough on the people who deliver it. We can expect a redress where the system will be more accommodating to physicians and value them more highly. For their part, physicians must understand that the world of health care is changing and should turn their energies to insuring that the best of our health care deliver system is preserved, thus helping to effect a new system that will well serve society's needs. What we're seeing now reflects an anti-institution and anti-establishment era, and I believe that we're going to work through that and sort out our priorities.

WHAT NEXT?

The stories have been told but the question persists, "What next?" This book does not present universal pronouncements about how to determine your direction in medicine and that was not to be expected. We must settle for hints and feelings. The challenge confronting a new medical graduate is in deciding how to make the most of a life in medicine and not trivialize it. The trick is to understand what "making the most" means, and you can't approach that by trial and error because you never get to relive the whole adventure. So, as many of the doctors in this book have said, you just do your best and try to arrive at reasonable compromises.

The stories given here provide an array of insights and each reader will take away something different from each story. If in the end the narratives serve as a springboard for further reflection, the project will have been justified.

Although the interviews reflect a certain amount of worry regarding the decline in the spirit and standards of clinical medicine caused by growing bureaucratic and legislative interventions, I find it heartening that just about everyone in the book had a good word for the practice of medicine as a way of life. And why not? The practice of medicine is inherently idealistic. In these cynical times, when dedication to others, aspirations to excellence, and acts of selflessness appear to have been devalued by indifference, idealism is still what medicine is all about. A good doctor must be far more than a bioscientific technician or a faceless minion in a bureaucratic health care corporation. A physician should be a caring friend to his or her patients as they cope with their personal afflictions and the occasional hardships and catastrophes of daily living.

341

The financial, administrative, and political aspects of medical practice are impinging greatly on the compassionate element of the physician's role, but that role is too essential not to endure. Compassion and caring on the part of the physician are important not only to the patient's well-being but to the physician's as well because over a lifetime those attributes make the doctor a better person.

Several themes recurred in the interviews. One is the need to know yourself and to be honest with yourself; but that is not easily achieved—it requires work, time, and integrity of purpose. Another theme relates to the close relationship between medicine and change. Today the pace of change in medical care is greater than ever for both the content of medicine—the basic scientific knowledge, diagnostic and therapeutic technology, patterns of clinical care, and more—and the context of medicine—the economics, regulations, organization, and so forth. Even the patterns of disease are changing: witness AIDS, tuberculosis, and strep infections. Adapting to change and putting it to constructive use are inescapable imperatives in a physician's life. Occasionally all this change leads to a midcareer shift from one discipline to another. This can be a stimulating event even when it is precipitated by regrettable circumstances.

Conflicting demands abound in medicine, and coping with them requires mature and intelligent balancing. Many of the conflicts relate to time. For example, one of the basic gratifications of medical practice is taking the time to talk with patients, but the current economic and administrative restructuring of medicine has eroded the visiting time with patients and this creates an unfortunate dilemma for caring physicians. If medicine is to be a calling, as it was once regarded by many of its practitioners, then it will demand so much of a physician's time that it will conflict with time for family, inner self, and a life beyond medicine.

Another growing conflict derives from the fact that physicians are trained to be advocates for each patient's best interests, but too often in practice today physicians are pressured to look to the greater good of a budget—even if it means abandoning the traditional role as patient advocate. Many doctors went into medicine to serve people at a level that transcends financial considerations, yet such considerations are now in the ascendancy and often predominate in the form of cost containment measures that pit the best patient care against the least costly patient care.

Contending with mixed messages is another issue in a doctor's life. Thus:

- Society calls for more primary care physicians but directs its rewards and plaudits to the specialists. Medical specialists are cast as cold and unfeeling clinicians by some patients and as overutilized economic burdens by some administrators, but the flow of new knowledge and new technology only increases the demand and the need for specialists, even superspecialists.

- Society wants physicians to be more humane and caring, but it accepts insurance systems that force patients to switch physicians at almost regular intervals thereby undermining the human relationship between doctor and patient.

- Society wants to contain the costs of medical care by decreasing access to high-technology tests and treatments, but when someone becomes sick the demand is for the best and newest regardless of cost.

- Society wants good health for everyone but too many people persist in their medically self-destructive personal habits.

- Society wants ready answers to its medical problems; however, laboratory researchers are revealing the boundless complexities of disease mechanisms and simple answers are hard to come by.

- Society wants more medical research accomplishments but makes it difficult and even professionally unattractive for physicians to become clinical investigators.

A physician works in an environment roiled by these and many other contradictions and must learn to manage them.

Stress abounds in a physician's life. For some it is the stress of life-and-death decision making. For others it is the nagging stress of the avalanche of petty bureaucratic demands on their time and attention. For still others it is the stress of marching to the beat of the demands of academic advancement while trying to remain a concerned physician and a generous teacher. And for others it is the stress of failed expectations, disappointments, or flawed career decisions. Osler was right about the need for equanimity in a doctor's life.

All this being so, why become a physician? Because, as one of the interviewees said, "It is still a most honorable profession." The unparalleled privilege of serving the profound needs of patients of all kinds, the opportunity for personal growth, the excitement of the rush of new insights to neuroscience, genetic disorders, mechanisms of malignant transformation, and on and on—all of these make medicine an attractive career. The difficulties are to be recognized and dealt with. Recent medical graduates say that never having known the halcyon days bemoaned by their seniors makes it easier for them to surmount the problems in today's medical setting. Carving a professional niche in this setting is challenging but need not be daunting.

To those readers who are not physicians but who have read this book out of curiosity about what goes into the shaping of a doctor or who seek a bit of guidance in planning their own careers, I hope your interests have been served. To medical graduates just starting out, or to more mature physicians contemplating a career change, I hope these stories have been interesting and helpful. To all readers, I wish you good fortune and, appropriately enough, good health.